Lesley Ackland with Malu Halasa

Pilates Over 50

Longer, Leaner, Stronger, Younger

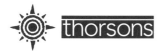

"It is never too late to be the person you could have been."

– George Eliot

Thorsons
An Imprint of HarperCollins*Publishers*
77–85 Fulham Palace Road,
Hammersmith, London W6 8JB

The website is www.thorsonselement.com

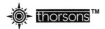

and *Thorsons* are trademarks of
HarperCollins*Publishers*

First published as *Pilates for a Fabulous Body* 2001
This revised edition published 2003

10 9 8 7 6 5 4 3 2

© Lesley Ackland and Malu Halasa 2001

Lesley Ackland and Malu Halasa assert the moral right
to be identified as the authors of this work

A catalogue record for this book is
available from the British Library

ISBN 0 00 715551 4

Photographs © Guy Hearn
Illustrations by Melanie Vandevelde

Printed and bound in Great Britain by
Martins The Printers Ltd, Berwick upon Tweed

Contents

A Letter to the Reader

Pilates is the perfect exercise regime for the over 50s, combining low-impact exercises with resistance training and weight-bearing exercise to build and maintain bone density, keep your joints flexible, your body supple and your mind active.

The exercises in this book are based on the ones that I myself use in my own exercise routine, which I have been doing for the last 15 years to create the body that I have, and that I'm happy with, in my late forties.

I take exercise seriously, because my job requires me to be very strong. I exercise for about an hour-and-a-half five or six times a week, using the specialized Pilates equipment in the studio and doing mat work exercises. I also go to a local gym three times a week. I make sure I alter my routine to suit the needs of my body at the time and my particular mood, which is one of the reasons that Pilates has kept my interest and enthusiasm over the years.

Although most of you will probably neither want nor be able to spend this amount of time exercising, doing the exercises in this book regularly a couple of times a week, together with an active lifestyle, will help make you feel leaner, stronger, fitter and younger.

If the only thing you take away from this book is opening out your shoulders, standing up straight and walking through your day with more energy and more enthusiasm, then I'll be very happy for you.

Lesley Ackland

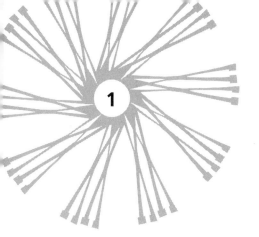

Introduction

Pilates Over 50 is a fitness manual for people in their fifties and sixties who, while leading moderately active lives, are keen to achieve and maintain a more toned and healthy body. As a 45 to 60-minute daily maintenance routine, *Pilates Over 50* is specifically designed to defeat the ageing process.

The effects of ageing are pernicious. Bad posture can lead to habitual back pain. A poorly aligned body can cause stiff neck and headaches, and even breathing problems. Aching joints can develop into crippling arthritis or rheumatism. As our bodies age, they have a tendency to become stiff and inflexible. In order to avoid the tight hamstrings, bent knees, round shoulders and forward-pointing neck that are the hallmarks of ageing, the exercises in *Pilates Over 50* will work your joints and mobilize your spine, to give you the fluidity of movement of someone much younger.

Drawing on the classic Pilates' principles of concentration and coordination, the exercises in this book will not only tone and strengthen your muscles (vital for helping combat diseases such as osteoporosis); they are designed to get you to focus on the correct use of exercise that will result in a streamlined body which will make you feel taller – just one of the many benefits of good posture that also include feeling upright, more focused and open. Through continual exercise and mobilization of your body, linked with a reasonably healthy lifestyle, I believe that the effects of ageing and gravity can be reversed.

The exercises in *Pilates Over 50* are the ones that I myself have been doing for the last 15 years. They've also been taught to and have benefited people who have come to my body-conditioning studio, Body Maintenance, in the Pineapple in London's Covent Garden.

THE SECRET OF PILATES

The secret of Pilates is that it doesn't build bulk. One of the most common problems I encounter in women who come to the studio is their lack of upper body strength. Strength is not bulk. It's easy to confuse the two since a lot of people nowadays lift heavy weights in the gym. Contrary to the idea behind most gym-based workouts, a huge amount of exercise can be accomplished without weights. When I was the advisor to the Birmingham Royal Ballet, I devised a 20-minute, 12-exercise programme that used nothing more than an alarm clock and a couple of pillows. Even without gym weights (or alarm clocks), you can increase body strength by using your *own* body weight and by working against gravity.

Instead of rushing into an exercise class and thrashing it out for an hour with a hundred other people, Pilates makes you stop and think about what you are doing. By focusing the mind, regulating your breathing and making use of internal resistance, the exercises in *Pilates Over 50* are more cerebral than other workouts that rely on rote alone, which of course has the added benefit of keeping the mind active and alert. You don't just have to learn a series of movements; you must also learn the concept.

Pilates employs a much more rounded exercise technique for both men and women. By expanding muscles, not bunching them up with exercise, they become longer and leaner. You will feel taller and trimmer and, as a result, completely at ease with your own body. Pilates produces a cosmetically beautiful body that is still strong enough to be useful.

The beauty of Pilates is that anyone, at any age, can do it. *Pilates Over 50* features strong muscle toning exercises to give you the sort of arms, shoulders, legs, abdominal muscles and buttocks on which clothes will hang beautifully, regardless of your size. Through the controlled, progressive and intelligent exercise regime featured here, you can totally reshape your body in the same way I did mine.

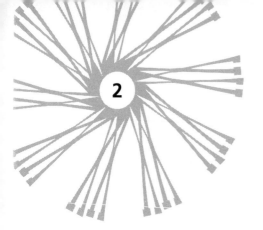

2

Discovering Pilates

In the 1980s, when exercise, body conditioning and aerobics were becoming popular, I realized that I didn't have an interest in my life outside my work as a teacher. So I decided to attend fitness classes in the old dance centre in Covent Garden, and found that I enjoyed them. Eventually I began to do teacher training in body conditioning. Around this time the first Pilates studio opened in the Pineapple, and I went to classes out of curiosity. Very quickly I realized that Pilates was the broadest exercise programme I had encountered; first, because it involved so many different complementary exercise techniques and, second, because its original basis in injury rehabilitation provided an intellectual basis behind the technique.

The system had been developed in the mid-1900s by German-born Joseph Pilates. Interned in Britain during the First World War, he devised a series of pulleys and weights to help rehabilitate injured soldiers. Using his exercise system, even hospitalized soldiers were able to prevent muscle wasting in healthy parts of their bodies. Back in Germany, the dancer and choreographer Rudolph von Laban incorporated Pilates' techniques of stretching and warm up into his own dance method.

In the 1920s, Joseph Pilates went to New York, set up a clinic and was soon helping injured ballet dancers. One of his greatest strengths was his ability to individualize exercise programmes, enabling dancers to work through their injuries, as well as increasing their stamina and strengthening their bodies. Through his low-impact exercise technique, dancers stayed in peak condition despite suffering from injuries. His success rate made him popular with such luminaries as George Balanchine, who was in charge of the New York City Ballet at that time, and dancer Martha Graham.

Pilates was a man before his time, writing about well-being as early as 1945 in his book *Return to Life Through Contrology* – the name he himself gave to his system.

*The acquirement and enjoyment of physical well-being, mental calm and spiritual peace are priceless to their possessors ... Self confidence follows. The Ancient Athenians wisely adopted as their own the Roman motto: '**Mens sana in corpore sano**' [A sound mind in a sound body].*

Pilates is a preventative exercise system. By correcting bad posture, it prevents injuries from developing later on in life. The best therapy for dancers, it soon became a favourite of Hollywood starlets, and over the past decade, a younger generation of celebrities, from Madonna to Uma Thurman, is starting to take advantage of its streamlining and realignment techniques.

For someone like myself, from a teaching and academic background, Pilates is the only discipline in the health and fitness field that offers both an intellectual challenge and the opportunity to draw on my existing skills. A distinct philosophy underpins the way in which Pilates' exercises have been developed and taught. First and foremost, it relies on a detailed knowledge of the body. Pilates also stresses that the exercises must evolve to keep pace with ever-changing bodies, even when that change is sudden and unforeseen. When I started teaching Pilates 15 years ago, I remember someone walking into one of my open classes, saying that they had just slipped two discs!

In a mat work class, you have to be quite strict about what exercises you allow an injured person to do (and you are limited by the group class situation). In my Body Maintenance studio, we actually see some people within 48 hours of surgery for rehabilitation treatment; sometimes they're still in plaster. The more obscure the injury the greater the challenge and, of course, no two injuries are the same. Ankles can strain in a hundred different ways. Everyone's needs are different, something that a body conditioning system like Pilates can take into consideration. It is this acknowledgement of how bodies work, change and age which makes it ideal for people later in life.

Throughout our lives, all of us have a natural ability to move and function well, but this can be hindered by habitual body patterns and by becoming what I call 'posturally trapped', i.e., droopy and less flexible as we get older! As the body ages, you need constantly to change and challenge it, and this process is different from person to person. Some of my clients find that they can exercise longer and harder as they grow older. For others, it may be that having a baby or suffering a serious injury – maybe a broken leg – has slowed them down or stopped their exercise programmes altogether. Bodies also have a tendency to show emotional and psychological changes like bereavements, stress or unemployment. In the Body Maintenance studio, some clients require individually designed exercises, and my expectations of what they are capable of doing varies from week to week. I have 70-year-old clients who still run to catch the bus, over-forties who can't lift a suitcase and 20-year-old dancers who, after injuring themselves, can't touch their toes. Exercises must be tailored to meet specific needs. This is the way I run the studio and this is the way that I have learned to choose exercises for myself.

While the core technique of Body Maintenance is Pilates-based, because of the philosophy underpinning the technique, I keep an open mind and have examined other exercise disciplines. For instance, I realized that a yoga stretch would be very useful for one of my clients and their body at a particular time. Sometimes I have enhanced a mainly Pilates programme by adding movements from physiotherapy, Feldenkrais, or postures from Alexander technique. I don't feel trapped or curtailed by an exercise regime I have been doing for 15 years, which means that I am free to change it. For me, openness to new ideas and disciplines has been one of the main benefits of the years I have spent teaching Pilates. Since every person's body presents a unique challenge, I haven't become stuck in the way that I want my clients – or myself – to exercise.

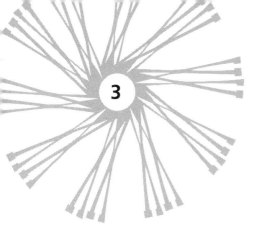

3

Fighting Ageing Through Exercise

In my late twenties, I had a crisis. I had always been the same size and then suddenly I started to put on weight. I tried to convince myself that it wasn't happening. I actually thought that my clothes were shrinking. Then I discovered Pilates and began to reshape my body.

Women get cleverer about exercise once they turn 30. They know from experience that getting hot and sweaty once a week in an aerobics class isn't going to have any long-term effects. The 1980s was a very conformist decade, and that went for exercise, too. Twenty years later, people are examining a wide range of body conditioning methods and deciding what's right for them at their particular time of life.

Now that I am in my forties, not only have I benefited from the physical effects of Pilates – better alignment of my body, toning and streamlining – but I have also benefited from the preventative aspects of doing the exercises: reduced aches and pains and the alleviation of stress and tension. Pilates has also helped me to recover more quickly when, for example, I strained my ankle running down the Pineapple stairs.

I realize that the amount of physical activity I accomplish daily is difficult for other people. If you have a desk-bound job, or if your job is not enjoyable, it is difficult to expend a lot of physical energy on a day-to-day basis. Gauging from the experience of many friends and clients, once they start working after college it becomes increasingly difficult for them to find the time to exercise. With increased commitments to work and home-life, this becomes harder over the years. So by the time they reach their forties and fifties, people find that their choices of career and lifestyle – raising children, eating hurriedly, having a sedentary job – have resulted in lower energy levels and a slower metabolism, which makes them more prone to weight gain.

There is no disputing this fact: the more stressed and upset we are, the more lethargic we feel. But the less we feel inclined to exercise, the more we actually need to. A lack of exercise results in tight muscles and underused joints. Bad posture starts to creep in from working all day in front of a computer or from sitting down all the time, whether in the office, on the underground or in a car. The tighter our bodies get, the more negative our body image becomes. The less mobility we have in our body, the worse our posture becomes – the tighter the ribcage, the rounder the shoulders, the more shallow the breathing. The blood doesn't pump so well around the body. We don't feel energized. We're not breathing oxygen in as a life force. We're not getting rid of toxins. So the incorporation of exercise into your daily routine is vital. As a lifestyle choice it will enable you to live better and longer if, at least twice a week, you go either to a Pilates studio or a gym, or for a swim, or for a two- or three-mile walk.

However, if you can't get to a Pilates studio, gym or a swimming pool, small changes can be made on a day-to-day basis. The first easy, but important one is to utilize your legs more. The more you walk, the more you take the stairs, the more energized you will feel, and the more you'll feel your heart and muscles working. If there is any one lesson to be learned from *Pilates Over 50*, it is to increase the amount of physical activity in your daily life, whether by small or large increments.

I am fortunate in that my life and work revolves around health. My morning begins with a 20-minute walk to the studio. I spend very little time sitting down, since my job demonstrating exercises is physically demanding. However, I am still able to find the time to exercise myself. Either before I begin teaching or after I've finished, I do an hour-and-a-half or so of exercise every day. I am also lucky to have a career that I like – even though it took me until my thirties to discover what it was! If you are in a negative working environment, it is doubly difficult to change your mindset or your occupation to force   yourself to become more physically active. However, there are less radical solutions than changing your job. You can incorporate more physical activity into your work and leisure time on a day-to-day basis.

The exercises outlined in *Pilates Over 50* are the ones I myself do five or six times a week. Many people would say that I exercise very seriously. But this is what I've had to do to achieve a body at my age that I am very comfortable and happy with. The most important conclusion to come to after reading and trying the exercises here is that everyone, no matter what their occupation or age, can find about 45 minutes or some kind of free time for physical activity. Maybe at the beginning it is only at the weekends. Afterwards you can focus on what you can do to activate your body on a day-to-day basis. Pilates may not be the fountain of youth. However, the exercises and the lifestyle advice will make you feel better and younger.

BODY TYPES

Defying the ageing process greatly depends on individual characteristics and habits. There is no easy formula, but with the right exercise, eating and drinking sensibly, and positive outlook, it is not impossible. Obviously part of who and what you are depends on your genetic inheritance. Sometimes this is an added bonus and sometimes it is not. When it isn't, it shouldn't be looked upon as an insurmountable hurdle. Because of my parents, I tend to look youthful. I come from a family that doesn't age dramatically, partly because we don't put on very much weight, and partly because none of us likes sitting in the sun. My mother is extremely fit and healthy for a woman her age. She runs her own business and has a very positive mental outlook, as well as a very active physical life. She runs up and down three flights of stairs all day and organizes a highly successful enterprise with a large staff. While most women her age would have retired 20 years ago, she won't consider it. She looks very youthful and has kept her figure.

WEIGHT, METABOLISM AND ATTITUDE

The first rule about your body is that you have to be happy with your weight. If you're happy with how you look, then you are obviously comfortable with who you are. If you are not happy, then it's a problem. It is essential to be comfortable with your own body – whatever its size. However, I will say that being underweight or overweight for your age has a detrimental effect on your body's ability to cope with the effects of ageing. I won't theorize about what 'underweight' is, because to quantify it, height and body types have to be taken into account, but I do see a lot of people who are underweight – people who are painfully thin for their age and body type – who complain about spinal, hormonal and emotional problems. These problems are very often directly related to excessive slimness, which causes difficulties with bone density and affects joint mobility.

Everyone understands the problems of being overweight: you may suffer from swollen ankles, have difficulty walking, even get out of breath climbing up the stairs. These sorts of things interfere with a normal lifestyle. If you get out of breath leaning down to play with your grandchildren, you're putting excessive damage on your internal organs, muscular system and your blood pressure. Severe problems with weight cause pressure on the joints. If your weight causes dizziness, fatigue, or even exhaustion, you can't lead a normal life.

If any of this relates to you, a sensible medical overview is essential to enjoying life as much as possible. We have the medical technology to ensure we can survive longer but there is no point having longevity if our quality of life is not good and we suffer chronic aches and pains.

As you get older, if your weight is causing you physical problems, then it is something that must be addressed. As we age our metabolism slows down, so we have to work harder to burn up the same amount of energy. Alternatively, we have to change to an energy source that is more easily digestible – in other words less fats and sugars in our diet. We also have to start adopting a healthier lifestyle that is more suited to our age and to a slower metabolism.

Controlled by the pituitary gland, metabolism is the complex and delicate process of burning energy to maintain a healthy body. The speed at which your body can use up the energy available to it is called the Basal Metabolic Rate (BMR), and it is determined by a chemical compound called adenosine triphosphate.

Metabolic processes in humans can be divided into two areas: anabolism and catabolism. Anabolism, or constructive metabolism, is the process of using energy to create new cells and to maintain existing ones. Catabolism, or destructive metabolism, governs the cycles of energy around the body so that body temperature can be maintained and complex chemical units be broken down into smaller substances, which are then excreted from the body through the kidneys, intestines, lungs and skin. When anabolism exceeds catabolism, growth or weight gain occurs.

Therefore figuring out your body's metabolic rate is important when you start an exercise or dietary programme. You will be more in touch with your body if you can respond to and predict its energy requirements. But this is not an easy thing to do. On the one hand metabolism is a deeply personal subject, genetically pre-programmed. On the other, it is also determined by environmental, social and lifestyle factors.

Thus, the things that can affect your metabolic rate are manifold, and you should learn which you can manipulate, and which you have to live with. It is also essential to realize that a fast metabolic rate isn't necessarily a good thing. Fast energy burners – who are usually thin – pay for their figures with fatigue, depleted mineral stores, moodiness, and an impaired ability to concentrate. Conversely, slow energy burners are more vulnerable to hyper-insulinism, insomnia, heart disease and diabetes. The key is to find a natural and healthy level that is right for you. Listen to your body.

Some factors affecting BMR can be changed; others can't. For example, women tend to have a slower metabolic rate – meaning that the turnover of energy takes longer and calories take longer to burn off – than men, since they usually, naturally, have more body fat. Inconsistent sleep patterns can also affect your BMR. Too much sleep will slow it down; too little will speed it up. Smoking accelerates BMR by 10 per cent – but it is definitely not a healthy way of keeping weight off, just as going without sleep isn't either!

The only way of increasing your BMR in a healthy, controlled way is through paying attention to your lifestyle and your diet. Avoiding sugary foods is just as important as avoiding fatty foods. If you have those mid-afternoon energy slumps, it is because you are experiencing a drop in blood sugar, resulting in fatigue. You can avoid fluctuations in your blood sugar and stabilize your metabolism by choosing meals rich in protein mixed with complex carbohydrates and a small amount of healthy fats. This will create a steady flow of blood sugar.

Even more essential than diet is your lifestyle. Exercise equals energy. Building more muscle – not necessarily bigger muscles, but stronger, toned, more efficient muscles to replace fat – will increase your resting metabolic rate, and lead to a higher caloric usage and more overall energy. So, as I have said before, making minor adjustments to your lifestyle – taking the stairs instead of the lift – can fundamentally change the natural balance of your body and improve your health.

Personally, I have taken steps to make sure that my metabolism does not slow down. If anything, it has speeded up. I keep it running by a combination of exercise and a positive outlook. I also make a point of not allowing myself to be psychologically influenced by concepts of ageing. I'm not saying they're not true, but I feel it is counter-productive to pay attention to them. So I don't. I'm a great believer in the idea that you have to keep stretching yourself, in terms of your life and your career. People need to take on new challenges. By stimulating your intellect and learning about new ideas and concepts, the mind as well as the body is invigorated. This is the real secret to keeping young.

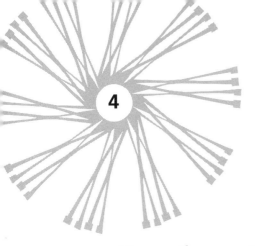

4

Delaying Ageing Through Correct Diet

It is extremely important to balance exercise with the kinds of foods you eat. 'Diet' is an overloaded and overused concept. What we should and shouldn't eat, how the famous get thin, how they stay thin, are media myths that have pushed many of my clients to dive for the nearest chocolate bar or doughnut.

As adults we should give up eating the sugary sweets and salty snacks that children do and develop an adult palate. We need to move away from nursery food to a wide range of nourishing and enjoyable adult foods. If national character is revealed through eating habits, Americans and the English have a tendency to chew on the run or eat at their desks. Lunchtime favourites are sandwiches or other quick snacks, which can be consumed with a minimum amount of fuss in the minimum amount of time. In the UK, food tends to be eaten as quickly as possible, while many leisurely hours are spent drinking and socializing in the pub. This attitude towards food and drink contrasts greatly with that in bars on the Continent, where they often serve some kind of appetizer with alcohol – something that's rarely taken in isolation.

In Spain and in Italy, for example, families make the time to sit down together and enjoy a proper meal. Not only is the European schedule of eating healthier than the Anglo-Saxon one – their main meal in the afternoon leaves ample time to burn calories – they have a more leisurely attitude toward food. They don't count the calories or watch their cholesterol, and tend to use ingredients that are known for their healthiness. Compared to English and American national dishes, the foods that characterize a Mediterranean diet have been shown to be healthy and good for promoting longevity.

An important reason not to over-eat is because of the pressure it puts on your digestive system. As we get older, some foods become harder to digest. Personally I don't eat meat, but that's an individual preference. I also don't drink milk. After living so long without it, I'm sure I would have difficulty digesting it. Additionally, there are certain foods that make me feel less energized, and there are foods that give my face a puffy look or make me physically uncomfortable. The effects of different foods change from body to body. Often it is difficult to keep track of the effects of what we eat. For people who are prone to food allergies, it is a good idea to keep a diary of what you eat and when, to refer back to it if you have a reaction to something you ate.

Another important aspect of eating is that what we eat informs what we expect to eat. People who live on ready-made supermarket meals, which have a high fat content, automatically turn to that kind of food when they're hungry. However, if you make the necessary changes to your diet, eventually what you consider a feast will also change. Instead of crisps, you might reach for sushi.

Our expectations of food also are also related to our ability and willingness to regularly introduce new foods into our diets. I can remember, aged three, being taken by my father to a Chinese restaurant – which was still a novelty at the time, even in central London. I can also recall when avocados were first introduced into the country. For a long time British cuisine was baffled by the avocado. But eventually they were eaten in salads and made into guacamole. Healthy eating includes experiencing different kinds of foods you wouldn't normally try.

EVERYTHING IN MODERATION

Everyone is aware that we should cut down on fats and sugars. It is the same with caffeine and alcohol. It is all too easy to become a victim of over-eating and over-drinking. If you want to change, you must create an eating style that suits you. If you're living on cappuccinos, take-away pizzas and pastries then that's a problem – there's a huge imbalance in your diet. It is full of sugar and additives. If you haven't made that psychological leap to a healthier diet (and some people from a strictly fast-food background never do), now is the time to try. You will suddenly find that food is no longer an enemy but a friend. Instead of feeling that every time you eat, you are punishing yourself, your diet can become exciting, interesting and enjoyable.

It is vital to eat foods you enjoy. If you're going to put yourself on a particular eating regime with food you hate, then the change in your diet will not be a positive one. And this negative energy will reverberate into other aspects of your life.

Eat food that you enjoy, even if you eat smaller quantities of it, rather than persecute yourself by eating what is considered the 'perfect' regime. These rigorous diets are often too difficult and, moreover, they're not actually healthy. Exchanging a meal for a calorie-controlled drink is a mistake. Food is to be enjoyed – it is to be chewed.

The main consideration about food and diet is to do everything in moderation. Normally I don't enjoy sweet tasting foods. However, if I really crave something then I don't deny myself. In this way, I avoid building up frustrations about the way I want to look. Frustration, like low energy, is only counter-productive.

DRINKING: THE GOOD AND THE BAD

All the diet experts say you should drink lots of water. I drink between two and three litres a day. It is important for me, because of the amount of exercise I take. It also nourishes me and keeps my skin clear.

From personal experience I know that as I get older, it is harder and harder for me to metabolize alcohol, even in small quantities. If I'm going to be photographed for some promotional material, for example, it is a mistake for me to drink a glass of wine the day before, because the effects can be seen on my face. However, there are certain types of alcohol that complement different kinds of meals, and these should be enjoyed.

When I do drink, I know that alcohol will slow me down the next day and I won't have the same positive energy. Since the age of 40, I have become careful not to drink too much. Of course, there are ways around this: for example by drinking equal amounts of water to alcohol. Obviously a glass of wine with a meal can be pleasurable, but if you're starting to feel that alcohol is affecting you physically, then you should sensibly reduce your intake.

To summarize: for someone over 50, it is vital to cut down on fats and sugars in your diet. Take a look at your caffeine and alcohol consumption; drink more water; keep your face out of the sun and invest in yourself. Take care of yourself and by applying a sensible, disciplined approach to looking the best you can for as long as you can, you will enjoy your life and vitality for many years to come.

VITAMINS AND MINERALS: TO SUPPLEMENT OR NOT?

While everyone knows that vitamins and minerals are a vital part of a healthy diet, there has been an enormous amount of research, writing and debate about vitamin and mineral supplements. While they work for me, they may not work for you. I use them because my diet doesn't include meat, calcium or iron-enriched foods. So it is important for me to supplement my diet. Vitamin and mineral supplements are a personal decision that should be discussed with an expert – either your doctor or a qualified nutritionist.

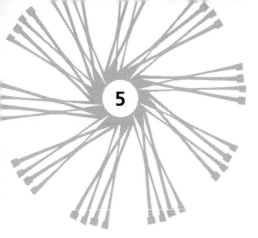

5

Pilates' Special Benefits for People Over 50

It *is* possible to maintain a healthy body – and by that I mean healthy joints, ligaments, bones and muscles, and an upright posture – well into your fifties and sixties, and even into your seventies and later, as some of my clients prove! You can also successfully defy a lot of the negative effects of ageing, caused by gravity, bad posture and the variety of problems that afflict especially women in later life. These problems are largely associated with the fact that we are living longer and longer, and we are fighting a battle against biology to do so.

I teach many people in my studio – from those in their late thirties through to a 90-year-old. Many women come to me after they have had a baby, discover that they like Pilates, and stick with it. There are a lot of very successful techniques I use to maintain women's health and fitness into later life, which are specific to what I do in Body Maintenance. Though these techniques are Pilates-based, many of the exercises and mental concepts we use are quite different to what you encounter in other exercise regimes.

The majority of my clients in their fifties are extremely fit and flexible, because in Body Maintenance we do an equal amount of strengthening and lengthening plus weight-bearing exercises to reverse the effects of ageing and gravity.

I teach people in their seventies and they tell me that they can do more press ups than their children in their forties who don't come to the studio. That's really heartening. The older my clients are, the more determined they are. They are less likely to say, 'It's too hot', 'I'm too tired', 'I can't come' – all the excuses some of my younger clients give. The older ones will make an effort to come regularly to the studio because they are determined to have an excellent quality of life for as long as possible.

* * *

There are three main areas that make Pilates an especially good exercise programme for mature people: countering the effects of osteoporosis, improving balance, and improving the pelvic floor muscles. A lot of

Pilates' exercises counter *lack of bone density and the effects of osteoporosis*. Everyone's skeletal mass starts to decrease in their forties or fifties. Osteoporosis is a more serious thinning of the bones. It is found most frequently in older women, when it is known as 'postmenopausal osteoporosis'. Factors that can accelerate the disease include inadequate physical activity, prolonged illness and a bad diet; it can also be hereditary.

Simple weight-bearing activities like walking up and down the stairs and carrying shopping bags can help to prevent osteoporosis. Pilates does do a lot of lower limb weight-bearing work to prevent and even help stabilize the disease. The most essential part of Pilates is taking the philosophy home. I encourage all my clients to be as active as possible. Interestingly enough, those with stairs in their house seem to have fewer problems than those who don't – walking up the stairs, and walking up escalators as much as possible, improves your weight-bearing capacity through all the lower body bones – the feet, the legs, the hips, etc.

For a lot of mature people intense cardiovascular exercise is not a good idea, because of the stress it places on the body. So I don't suggest to my 70-year-old client that she go on a treadmill. Because it is non-weight bearing, swimming is the best way for a lot of elderly people to tone up the body and improve cardiovascular health. But the fact that swimming is not weight bearing means that it's not enough of an exercise regime on its own. Although it is a fantastic exercise, it will do nothing for your bones. So walking is essential. However, walking and other lower-body exercises do not deal with problems related to osteoporosis and lack of bone density in the upper body.

In the studio, I concentrate on upper bodywork too. All of my clients do press-ups, and the techniques are demonstrated on pages 121, 122 and 128, and I recommend press-ups to everyone. However, not all my clients can execute full press-ups. Some do them with their knees on the ground, as you can see from page 121. If this is too difficult for you, start doing press-ups against the wall – this is still a useful weight-bearing exercise. Stand around a metre away from the wall; place your palms on the wall and do basic press-ups, breathing in as you lean towards the wall, and breathing out as you push away.

Don't hit your head on the wall! If you are too close to the wall, nothing will happen, but if your heels come off the ground then you're too far away. Don't arch your back either, and have your tummy tucked in.

Press-ups – however they're done – strengthen all the bones in the hands, wrists, forearms, elbows and shoulders. They will also help strengthen your upper back. One 78-year-old client still does her press-ups on her hands and knees every time she comes to the studio. A 90-year-old client does them leaning against the wall because her sense of balance is not what it was five years ago. But there's no way that she is going to stop doing press-ups. Recently I asked if she wanted to use the lift up to the studio and she looked horrified at the thought! There was no way that she wasn't going to climb those flights of stairs. The more stairs you climb, the better the bone density in the body.

This of course links back to a healthy diet and an active lifestyle. If you don't have a healthy diet and maintain an insufficient intake of nutrients, you will not be able to maintain the quality of bone structure that you need.

* * *

Another area linked to ageing is *proprioceptional balance*. This is the interaction between the nervous system and the muscles, tendons, ligaments and joints, which tells us how to react to our environment without necessarily needing to look and think out movements consciously. For example, when we walk on an uneven pavement, this proprioceptive input to the brain is subconsciously processed to allow the correct 'reflex' response to an input: the body quickly tells the brain that the ground is unsteady; the brain then sends messages to the muscles to prevent you from falling. Musculoskeletal injury may affect proprioception – as does old age. Poor proprioception combined with osteoporosis makes you vulnerable to broken bones when you fall over.

Unfortunately, we all tend to lose our sense of balance as we get older, and as a result we are more afraid of falling and breaking bones. We feel more vulnerable, particularly in a society that appears to be constantly rushing about, oblivious to others around, and that doesn't seem to value age. There is a general lack of respect for the physical demands of old age, as well as the simple lack of innate respect for people just as people.

For anybody over the age of 50, balance is something that tends to deteriorate, so it's important to do proprioceptive exercises. Some of my clients do a huge amount of balance exercises in the studio involving balance pads and wobble boards; these are not included here because they require specialist equipment. However, there is a simple balance exercise that most of my mature clients do – and a lot of my younger clients who have suffered any sort of injury or who have very bad postural problem: bad balance is not necessarily an age-related problem.

Balancing on one leg, both with eyes open and eyes closed, can be extremely difficult for some people. It can be made even more difficult by changing the surface on which you stand – by using a towel, for example. It's always better to do balance exercises in bare feet. The more you can walk round your house or your garden in bare feet, the more you will exercise the muscles in your feet, which don't tend to be used nearly so much when wearing shoes. Foot problems are again associated with age, due to stiffness and tightness. Taking care of your feet is essential and I can't emphasise it enough; there are as many bones in one foot as there are in the rest of your body.

Standing on One Leg

Stand with both feet grounded into the floor, with your weight equally distributed over your feet, head floating, and arms at your sides, tailbone dropped. Shoulders and neck are relaxed; the arms are hanging naturally in front of the body.

Don't rock forwards or backwards. Don't cling onto the floor with your toes. Very gently float one foot off the ground, hold for 10 seconds and put it down. Repeat four times, alternating your feet. Then do the same exercise with your eyes closed.

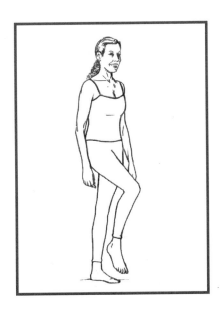

When you lift your leg, make sure the pelvis is not distorted and the hips remain level.

*   *   *

I can't stress how important it is to reverse the effects of gravity pulling us forward – the forward pointing chin, the rounded shoulders, the fear of falling, all of which starts to create a stooping posture. This is not totally age-related, but it can deteriorate with age, as people become more aware of their physical limitations and more concerned about the hustle and bustle of everyday life.

This brings me to the third area that Pilates is particularly good for – the *pelvic floor*. The pelvic floor is the group of muscles that sits in the bottom of the pelvis, often described as a 'sling', which supports the contents of the pelvic and abdominal cavity. The pelvic floor helps to maintain continence; it also plays an important role in preventing and treating lower back pain, and it helps to stabilize the pelvis.

Pelvic floor dysfunction can occur through childbirth, advancing age, long-term constipation and back pain. A third of all women over a certain age have some sort of stress incontinence caused by weakness in the pelvic floor muscles. But this is not something that tends to be discussed, because it is considered embarrassing. As we get older, muscles get slacker and don't function as well. Research and clinical findings indicate that the pelvic floor and deep abdominal muscle (the transverses abdominus) work together as a unit to help prevent lower back pain, sacroiliac joint problems and to prevent urinary leakage. The basic core stability contraction in Pilates works these muscles together.

All my clients, of any age, do pelvic floor exercises. After childbirth they are essential. After multiple births, they are more than essential. It is only in the last few years that people have become aware of how widespread pelvic floor problems are, because we are living longer and we are becoming less worried about talking about these problems and keeping them hidden. If you can't run for the bus, if you can't sneeze with confidence, if you're constantly worried about where the nearest toilet is, you need to

work on these issues. It's important to seek sympathetic medical advice –
whether it's from a specialist in this field, a doctor or a physiotherapist –
to check there isn't anything major going wrong. If there are no major
physical problems, it is purely a case of relearning to use these muscles
groups so they tone themselves up and you can go through life without
worrying where the nearest toilet is.

The pelvic floor exercises included here involve squeezing a small folded
towel, lying on your back, and fanning out the lower abdominal muscles.
You've got to think about the pelvic floor muscles and the transverse
abdominus, which runs diagonally between your two hip bones, between
your pubic bones and your navel. Most people spend their lives exercising
their rectus abdominus, the muscle that runs up the front, which gets a lot
of exercise anyway anytime you lean forwards or backwards. The lower
abdominals, the transversus, has to be actively worked on and consciously
thought about it. The pelvic floor muscles require a lot of mental
direction. It's a relearning process. Any sort of intervention in that area
will cause loss of function and dysfunction. To retrain these muscles is a

neuromuscular process and I cannot stress how important it is to exercise your internal muscles – to draw the external muscles in – rather than working the other way around.

In my studio, you will hear me screaming 'VAGINAL CONTRACTION!' with alarming regularity, and none of us are embarrassed. My clients have got the age where they're not worried about saying anything. What we're worried about is thinking can I sneeze? Can I laugh? Can I cough? Can I actually run for the bus? (And by run I don't mean sprint. For many people even a simple acceleration is out of the question.)

If this rings a bell with you, then do the exercises below, particularly the squeezing of the towel and the fanning. If you are really having problems, invest some money in some serious professional help after a proper medical check-up, be it a good local Pilates teacher or a well-trained physiotherapist. It's not embarrassing; it's a fact of life. Have a coffee morning. Sit round with your close friends of the same age, and ask how many of them are secretly having the same problem that you think is too embarrassing to talk about.

Preparing for Abdominal Exercises

You need to wake up your stomach muscles before you start exercising.
Lie on a towel or a mat with a relaxed back and a long neck, without
tucking the pelvis under. Take either a small cushion or a folded towel
and place it between your thighs.

Very gently breathe through your nose. As you breathe out, feel your
stomach muscles pulling down to the floor. Think of them pulling up and
into your spine. Hold your breath and count to four, at the same time
contracting your internal vaginal muscles. Breathe out slowly and relax
your muscles. You can count out your fingers on your stomach if you wish
so that you can feel the muscles you are working.

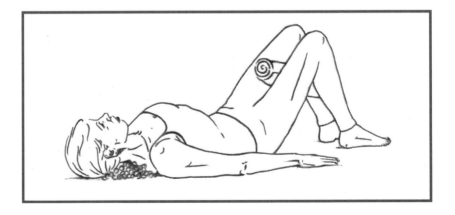

If you have high blood pressure, it is important that you do not hold your breath. Instead, breathe in slowly for a count of four, contracting your vaginal muscles, and then breathe out for a count of four as you relax your muscles.

As you breathe in through your nose, feel your stomach gently expand into your fingers. As you breathe out, feel your stomach pull away from your fingers. Feel your lower abdominal muscles working. Think of working on the transverse and the rectus abdominis muscles first, and the obliques second. Repeat this 10 times.

Working the Lower Abdominal Muscles (Fanning)

Lie in the same position, with your knees bent. You can place your hands on your hipbones. This helps to stabilize your pelvis. Begin with the right leg and open your right knee sideways. As you breathe out feel the resistance. Bring the leg back to the other one – breathing out and pulling your stomach in. Change legs. Now, breathing in, open the left leg to the side. Exhale and slowly close. Repeat 10 times, alternating legs each time.

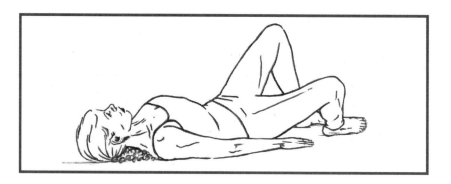

Don't tilt your pelvis and don't press your back into the mat.

In this exercise you can imagine the transverse abdominus muscle as a fan. When you breathe in and open your leg to the side, imagine a fan opening. As you breathe out, close the 'fan' up again, feeling the muscle tightening on its diagonal plane between your hip bones.

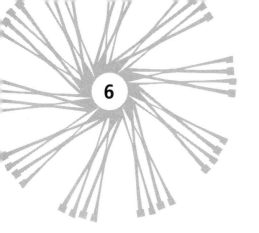

6

How to Use
Pilates Over 50

Modern lifestyles can polarize the attention we pay to our bodies. We may be obsessed with going to the gym for a month or so, and then neglect exercise altogether due to a simple lack of time. I am fortunate in that my lifestyle is always an active one; but for those who don't have as much opportunity to exercise, there are many ways in which these Pilates exercises can be woven into your everyday life.

CORE ESSENTIALS

Concentration

Pilates is an exercise regime like no other. It is often difficult for people to accept that they won't be doing a 60-minute Step Class or that they won't be sweating and straining with high resistance exercises. Pilates starts off slowly and gently, but it requires supreme mental and physical focus. To achieve this, you need to create time and space in your life where you can concentrate on the exercises, where you know you won't be interrupted. Obviously a specialized studio is the ideal place for Pilates, but if you can't get to one find an area in your house that you can transform into your Pilates sanctuary.

Equipment

The basic exercises I do every day require little or no equipment, so it is easy to do them at home. I usually exercise in front of a mirror so I can see what my body is doing, and so I can correct my posture and watch the progress I make in my exercises. It is good to exercise on a synthetic mat (something like a yoga mat is ideal, about 1.5m by 2m) so that your limbs are protected from bruising on a hard floor. A folded blanket can work just as well as a specialized exercise mat. In some of the exercises I hold weights – but if you don't have weights, use a can of beans, or something heavier if you're feeling strong. Sometimes I use a chair for support; make sure it is firm on the ground and won't slip away from you. The most advanced piece of equipment I use is a Dynaband – a long piece of elasticated rubber used by physiotherapists and readily available in health and fitness stores. Dynabands come in different colours, coded according to their resistance strength. I suggest that you use a blue Dynaband, which is a medium resistance band.

Clothes

I usually wear a body and loose tracksuit pants when I exercise, because it is important to have support and flexibility at the same time. The clothes you wear for Pilates must not restrict your movement at all. Natural fibres such as cotton are ideal because they keep you cool. Take off any dangling jewellery, and take off your socks so that you can feel the ground in touch with your feet.

Safety

Listen to your body when you exercise. Pilates is not about straining and sweating. If something hurts, stop, and try to figure out why. It is important to remember these points:

- Stretch your muscles after the more strenuous strengthening exercises
- Build up each exercise slowly and systematically
- Drink plenty of water before exercising, and re-hydrate when you've finished
- When trying new exercises, take them one step at a time
- If at any point you feel breathless, nauseous, chest pains (especially if accompanied by arm, neck, and shoulder pain), back pain, or if your muscles shake, then STOP immediately.

GUIDING PRINCIPLES

Pilates is a very precise form of exercise. It is different from other fitness regimes in that it requires a bit of groundwork. You should understand the six basic principles underpinning Pilates before you start.

1. Breathing

I try always to be acutely aware of the strong connection that exists between breathing and movement. This is something that is addressed in dance but no so much in the gym. For most Pilates exercises, you should breathe out on the point of effort. During the exercises think of your breath as a rejuvenating life force. If there is a tight area that is being stretched open for the first time, breathe into that new space – breath is a form of liberation, working the body from the inside out.

Oxygen nourishes the body and the brain. It is important to breathe deeply and fully, past the upper chest and right down into the lower lobes. That way you can properly energize large areas of your body. Breathing properly is a spiritual exercise: it creates equilibrium. Use it to the full when you do Pilates.

2. Control

Control means using the correct parts of the body for each particular exercise. Many people, for example, think that they are using their abdominal muscles during an exercise when they are, in fact, straining their neck and shoulders or hip flexors. It is best to try to make each exercise efficient by focusing on a particular muscle group.

Control and precision are synonymous in Pilates. All the exercises should be done slowly, in a meditative fashion. Don't allow your mind to wander.

Proper control within each exercise means minimizing the stress and involvement of other parts of the body. The whole body should be used in proportion. It is preferable to do five repetitions of an exercise in a thoughtful and methodical way than to go through hundreds of inefficient, overly strenuous motions. When I do the pelvic tilts, for example, I try to feel each individual vertebra at a time. Pilates is about being sensitive to your body.

When using free-weights, you should be in control of the movement by thinking about internal resistance, rather than using your shoulders or snapping your elbows back and forth. Focus on the muscles you're using while making sure that the rest of your body is relaxed and aligned. People often make what is a simple exercise into something quite torturous, thus creating distortion, tension, and the inability to minimize the movements of other parts of their bodies. With concentration it is possible to gain almost as much benefit from an exercise without weights, by using the concept of internal resistance.

3. Centring

In many eastern religions, the centre of the body is not the heart, but the pelvis. Pilates similarly encourages the development of one strong, core area that controls the rest of the body and supplies it with energy. The core is that part of your body that is bounded by a continuous band around the bottom of your rib cage and across the line of your hip-bones. This is the centre of your body, where the most important stomach and back muscles are. These muscles support your internal organs and keep you upright. Your arms and legs are extensions from the centre.

If you have a strong centre then you'll have a strong back, which means you can walk, stand and run without discomfort and pain. If you have a bad back this is an indication that your centre is not strong enough. Originally, human beings were not designed to stand up straight. The only reason we stand up at all is due to the muscles around the centre. We are constantly fighting gravity pulling us forward. This explains why so many people have problems with their neck and shoulder muscles. We are basically defying nature and gravity by standing up straight.

4. Flow

Each exercise I do in this book should be done in a smooth, flowing, undulating way. There is no room in Pilates for any sharp, jarring movements, or quick, jerky actions – these are the total antithesis of everything we are trying to achieve.

Every motion originates from a strong centre and flows out from there in a slow, gentle, controlled fashion. This warms the muscles, causing them to lengthen and open up the spaces between each vertebra in the spine. This extends the body to create a longer, leaner shape.

5. Precision

Attention to detail is essential to ensure that each movement is working in the correct manner. Before you start an exercise sequence, read the instructions carefully. Make sure you are properly aligned and pay attention to the Watchpoints. This will ensure that you do not expend excess energy doing an exercise incorrectly.

6. Coordination

Children run naturally, but for most adults basic coordination is a major problem. Most of us have lost the ability to coordinate our bodies and minds into unified beings. We no longer have the sense of our feet being in contact with the earth. We've lost the feeling of the way breath moves naturally through the body. The aim of Pilates is to regain neuromuscular connection between the brain and body.

This reconnection is best illustrated when I teach people the foot exercises. I sometimes joke that the feet are very far away from the brain, so they are slow to obey. But consider people who have lost the use of their hands. They can often do the same things with their feet that others can do with their hands. We all have the capability to be in touch with every part of our body, but we don't normally use it. If you don't use something in your body, it atrophies. Therefore, if you don't use your physical sense of coordination, you lose that innate ability.

Some of these exercises are complex because they are based upon the introduction of a more complicated concept than simple physical movement. They are trying to reintroduce the mind to the body. If I ask my opposite arm and leg to do something at the same time, by coordinating the breath and using a strong centre, I should be able to achieve it. If I slip in the street, I am more likely to regain my balance than to lose it. When someone throws a bunch of keys at me, I can usually catch it. Because I have that neuromuscular connection between my mind and body, I can react spontaneously, and this is where the proprioceptive concept – the linking of mind and body – comes into play.

In Pilates, we try to recreate your body as a coordinated whole, rather than thinking about individual areas. Coordination is paramount to the way the exercises flow. Ideally you should use breath, coordination and precision to do a limited number of repetitions properly.

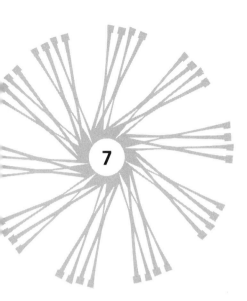

7

The Exercises

My previous books all concentrate on injury and rehabilitation, something that the Pilates technique is particularly good for. Yet, a little known secret about Pilates is that it is extremely dynamic for people who are already fit but who want to maintain that level of fitness and protect themselves against the physical effects of ageing. I don't give my clients exercises that I can't do myself – I feel it is important to lead from the front. Some of these exercises are included in here. They are exercises that I have been doing for the past 15 years. Executed with care and attention, they will give you good postural alignment, develop your strength and stability, and at the same time tone your body. The basic mat work starts with the spine, and soon moves into strengthening the centre. Even though I periodically change my programme, the exercises outlined below are the ones that I have found particularly beneficial in building not only the body, but one's own personal confidence.

* * *

The first sequence of exercises concentrates on warming up the spine and preparing the body for exercise, starting with the three classic Pilates rolling exercises. Then there are the mobility exercises for the hips and the ankles, which are interspersed with other routines. I see the entire pelvic tilt and abdominal sequence as working in conjunction with each other.

The rolling exercises and the pelvic tilts warm up and mobilize the spine in preparation for the abdominal exercises, so that your spine is relaxed into its neutral position and you're in the best anatomical position to work effectively. I exercise at least five times a week to achieve the desired results, although you don't have to do that much to benefit from Pilates!

This initial sequence also includes foot exercises because it is essential to feel grounded and in contact with the earth. You should be able to feel the flow of energy from the crown of your head down through the soles of your feet so you're not retaining tension in any of these parts of your body. The length and correct placement of your neck, the release of your spine and the softness of your feet are essential to achieve the body balance you require. In addition, focusing on equal weight distribution down both legs through the pelvic tilt will transform the imbalance we all have in our bodies, caused by standing incorrectly, sitting cross-legged or putting our weight on one leg.

The idea of these exercises is all about how to achieve, through visualization, the Pilates' principles of coordination, balance and centring. From this, the abdominal exercises flow naturally as you have now, hopefully, released the tension from these areas of your body. After the abdominals I like to do some standing work, because I can then really focus on recreating a correct standing posture from the correct prone posture I've just achieved on the floor. Because I've centred myself and worked my abdominals, I can now stand and do the exercises to warm up and mobilize my shoulders knowing that I'm in correct alignment and that I'm working my centre effectively.

Although the second sequence is the abdominals, I find it quite hard to separate the side stretches, the side lifts, the tricep lifts, the press-ups and the dips from working my centre. So I see the exercises from pages 115 to 126 as a continuation of my abdominal work.

When I've focused my mind on my abdominals, I move on from just working what people think are their stomach muscles to working on my side – using the obliques. With all the exercises in the sequence that involve lying on your side, you should be aiming to strengthen your entire upper body and the muscles in your back. You're also working towards the strong stabilization of the shoulder blades and the pelvis. These exercises are extremely challenging and I would never leave them out of my routine. I may not do them all every day, but I would do at least half of them.

Following on from the side stretch sequence are the press-ups and the dips. I like to do these after the side stretches because once I've focused on my centre, I then want to use that concentration to stabilize me as I strengthen my upper body. This sequence is also about correct alignment – the way the abdominals are controlling the exercise. It is not about how many I do, it is about how successfully I do them with correct postural alignment and core stability. So if I'm doing press-ups or dips I make sure I'm working evenly using both arms, because being right-sided, it is easy to lapse into working predominantly on that one side. I actively negate this tendency by concentrating on the positive Pilates' principles of core strength and coordination.

Rolling Up Like a Ball

Many people have little flexibility in their spines, so this exercise can be tricky.

First, sit holding your shins. From the photograph, you can see that I'm curled up like a ball. Then, as you breathe out, roll backwards as the stomach pulls in. Be careful not to roll too high up onto the neck. That way the upper spine doesn't get compressed. As you breathe in again, roll back up into the seated position. If you have trouble getting back up, use your arms to help to start off with.

Try to keep your heels close to your bottom and your shoulders relaxed. Do 10 repetitions.

 Watchpoint: Don't roll too far back onto the neck.

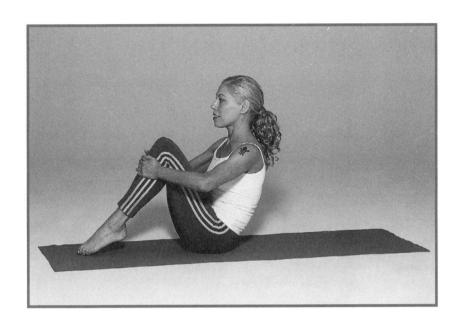

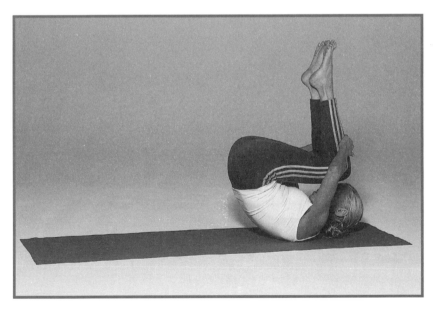

The Seal

Start in the same sitting position as *Rolling Up Like a Ball,* but with your

feet together and your knees apart. Your hands should hold onto the

outside of your ankles.

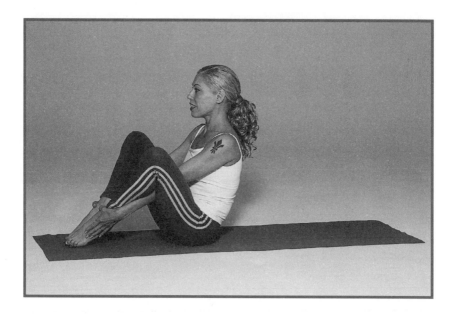

Sit up straight, resting on your toes. As you breathe out, roll backwards, but again, not too far up the neck. Lift back into the upright position on the inhalation. Repeat this rocking movement 10 times.

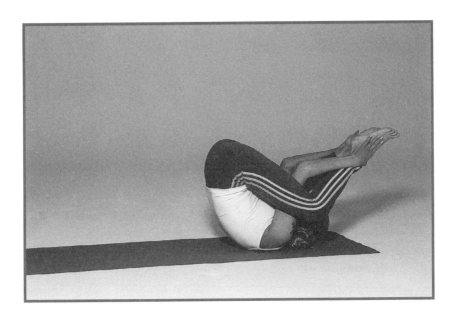

Open-Leg Rocker

Start in the same position as the *Seal*, with your feet together and your knees apart. Again, hold onto the outside of your ankles.

Make sure you are sitting up perfectly straight, then breathe in and straighten out both your legs. Breathe out and roll back (not too far up the neck), pause, breathe in, and balance. The balance is tricky. Breathe in again, bend your legs, and roll back to your starting position. Repeat this 10 times.

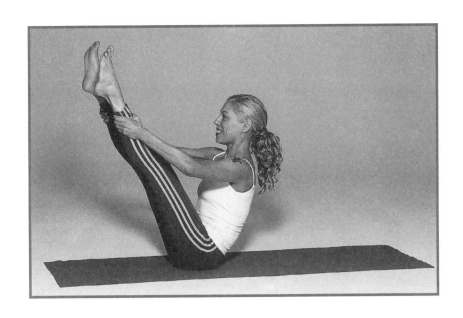

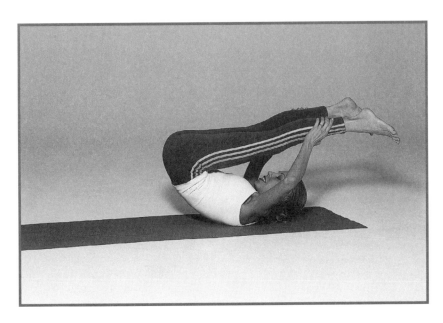

Roll out from the *Open-Leg Rocker* straight into the *Hip Rotation Exercise.*

 Watchpoint: If you have tight hamstrings and cannot straighten your knee, leave this exercise out of your routine.

Hip Rotation Exercise

This exercise helps to achieve greater flexibility and articulation in the hip sockets.

Lie down on a mat so that your tailbone is supported. Then bend your knees into your chest, holding onto your legs just below the knees. Your body should not move during this exercise and your head should be resting.

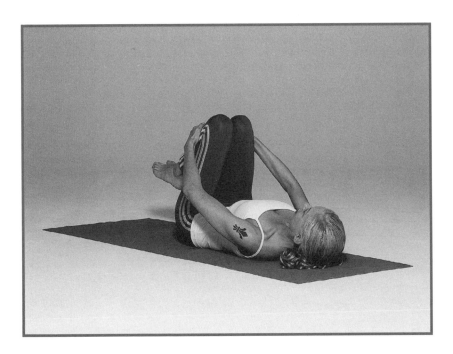

Open your legs so that your toes are together but your knees apart. Rotate your hips ten times in each direction. You should feel a passive stretch in your inner thigh, but this isn't the main point of the exercise. Feel the blood flow through your hips, your lower spine and pelvis warming up, and your hip sockets becoming more lubricated. This exercise is great for releasing tension in the hips.

Breathe normally, and make sure your legs are kept fairly close to your body. Do 10 rotations in each direction.

 Watchpoint: Hold onto the shins, never the knees.

Ankle Circles

This exercise relaxes the ankles, calves and feet.

Stay lying down and hold your legs up behind the thighs. Your feet and knees are together. Gently circle your ankles very slowly, taking six seconds to make a full circle in each direction. Do between six and eight repetitions in each direction.

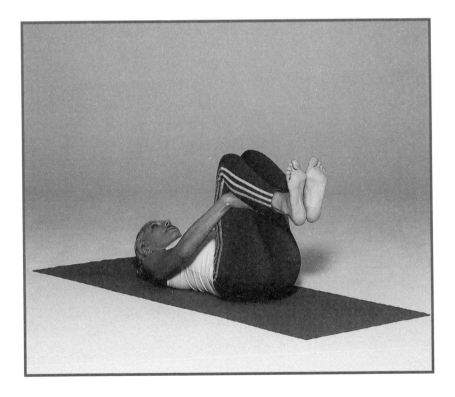

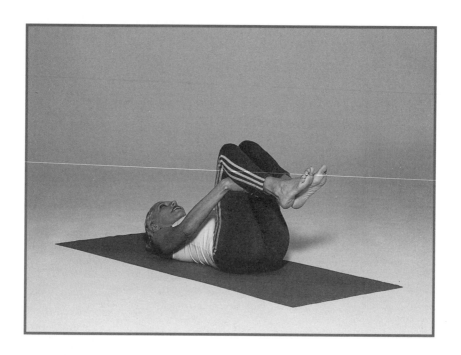

After the *Hip Rotation* and *Ankle Circles,* move into the *Pelvic Tilt* and the

abdominal sequence.

Pelvic Tilt

The Pelvic Tilt helps to warm up the back. Still lying on your back, your knees should be bent and your legs parallel, hip-width apart, feet flat on the floor. Place your arms by your side, and have your hands relaxed, flat, palm-down on the floor. This creates the correct alignment for the neck, shoulders, and upper body.

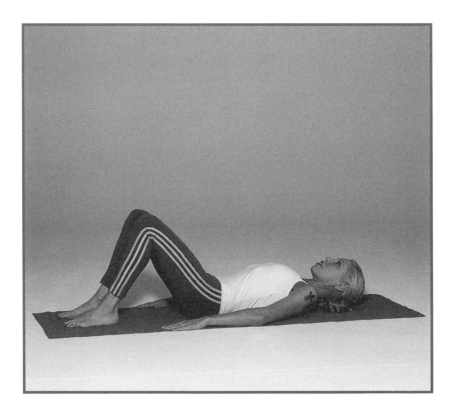

Breathe out as you tilt your pelvis forward and roll your lower back off the floor, one vertebra at a time. This makes for a great feeling of peeling your back off the floor. Only lift yourself up as high as your ribs remain relaxed and soft – don't push them forward. Make sure your chin doesn't tip backwards. This is the natural limit of spinal mobility.

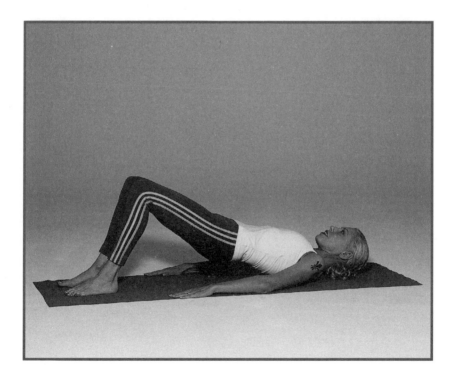

Then, gently breathing in, lift your arms over your head. Only take them as far back as your neck doesn't drop backwards. Reverse the movement as you breathe out, keeping your neck long as you roll down. Think of your sternum relaxing into the ground. The base of your spine should touch the floor last. Then bring your arms back to the starting position. Repeat the sequence 10 times.

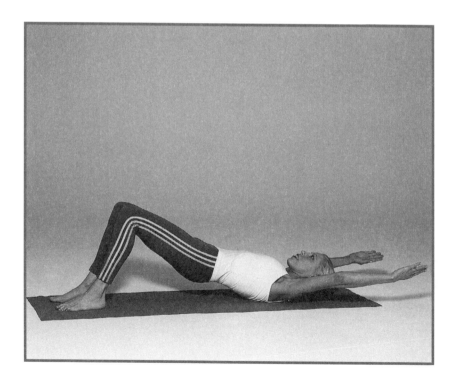

All the while the feet are firm but relaxed on the floor, and the toes are lengthening away from the body.

 Watchpoint: Don't try to flatten the back completely.

Pelvic Tilt with One Leg Crossed

This is the same exercise as the *Pelvic Tilt* except that you cross one leg over the other, with one foot remaining on the floor. Lift in the same way as before, alternating on each leg 10 times.

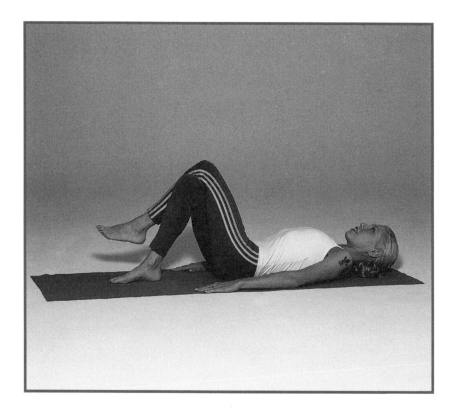

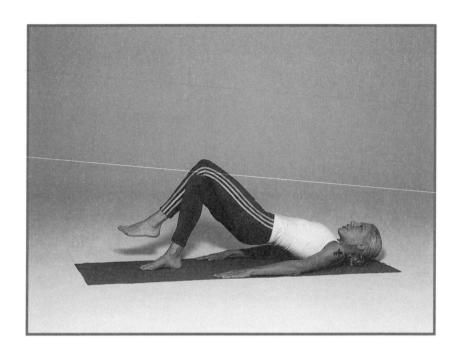

Pilates Over 50

Roll-Up

This exercise warms up the back and also stretches out all the tension in the hamstrings which builds up over the day.

Lie on your back with your legs straight in front of you, hip-width apart. The feet are flexed. Stretch your arms out behind your head, continuing the line you've made with your legs. Keep your middle back on the mat the entire time so that your arms aren't tempted to go too far back behind your head; don't arch your lower back.

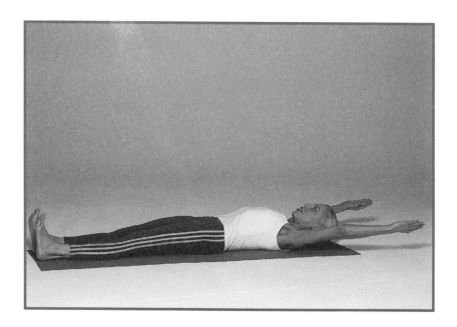

Breathing out, stretch your hands back over your head down to your thighs. Then, breathing in, lift your head, which should float naturally on top of your shoulders. On the next exhalation, use your abdominal muscles to curl the back up off the floor, one vertebra at a time, until you're in a seated position. Then lean forward a little more and stretch out your lower back and hamstrings. Breathe out and roll down to the floor. Repeat this movement 10 times.

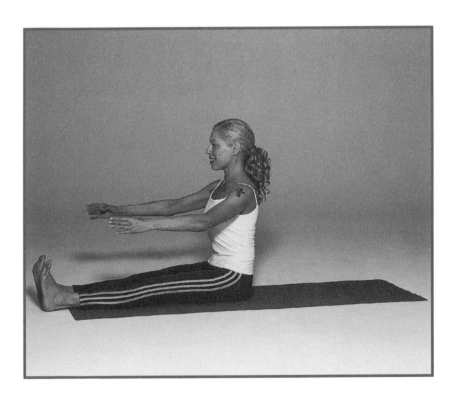

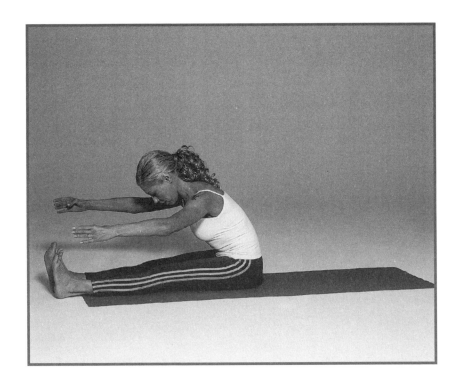

 Watchpoint: The energy goes through the heels, not through the front of the thighs. That way, you can engage the hamstrings as stabilizers.

❊ ❊ ❊

Now that you have warmed up your back and focused your mind, you're ready to move into the daily abdominal sequence, which includes all the *Side Lifts* and *Side Stretches*.

Basic Abdominal Curl

Lie on your back with your knees hip-width apart, as they were for the *Pelvic Tilt* exercise (page 77). Your hands are behind your head – but only for support, not to assist the abdominal muscles. You should be able to see your elbows out of the corner of each eye. Make sure your knees don't fan out.

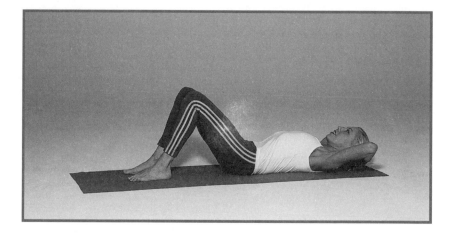

Breathing in through your nose, relax your abdomen and stare positively at the ceiling. Then, on the exhalation, lift your head and shoulders off the mat. Only lift as high as your stomach muscles flatten to your spine. This ensures a strong, flat stomach. I find it helpful to imagine a piece of string pulling me up from the pubic bone towards my navel. Your neck should always be relaxed: it is the stomach muscles that are doing the work.

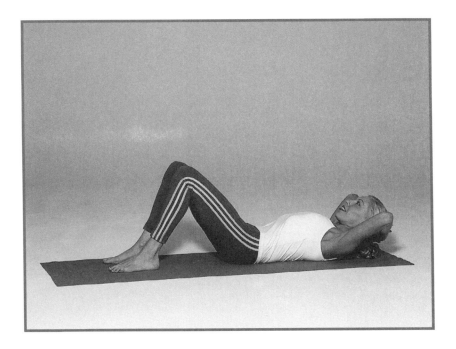

Try to feel all three sets of abdominal muscles going up and in, flattening and firming up. As you go down again, breathe in. Do 10 repetitions initially, but this is an exercise you can repeat up to five times during the mat-work sequence.

Watchpoint: Your head and neck float off the floor to maintain perfect posture throughout the exercise.

Single Leg Stretch

The next exercise in my sequence of abdominal stretches is a simple variation on the *Basic Abdominal Curl*.

Lying in the same position as before, with your hands interlaced behind your head, lift your head and shoulders slowly off the mat. As you exhale, extend your left leg down until it is a few inches off the floor. Breathing in, lower your head and replace the leg. Then breathe out and extend the right leg down, again until it is about an inch off the floor. Repeat this 10 times, alternating the legs.

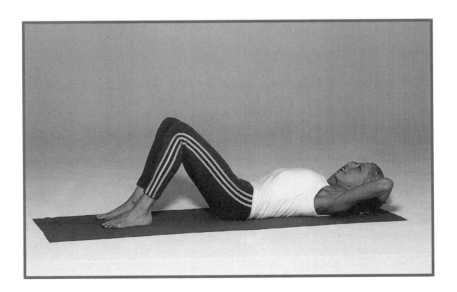

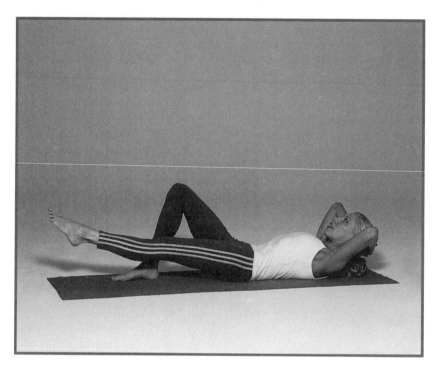

 Watchpoint: Make sure you exhale exactly as you curl forwards and not before.

Focusing on the same point on the ceiling helps the concentration and ensures that you don't pull your chin into your chest. That way you know you're not straining your neck or distorting your posture.

Abdominal Exercises

I do these three abdominal exercises every day. They are good for the lower abdominals and for pelvic stability. With all these abdominal exercises, try not to work the front of the thigh. Think of the hamstrings and the abdominal muscles doing all the work and the muscles in your legs lengthening. Make sure you don't grip your bottom. Start out in the basic *Pelvic Tilt* position, lying on your back with your arms beside you and your knees bent.

Abdominal Exercise 1

Lie on your back in the starting position, and be aware of your posture and the natural curve in your spine. There should be no contraction in the spine; your neck should be lengthening; your hips level; and your arms softly beside you. You might want to have a towel behind your head.

Breathing out, pull your stomach into your spine and extend one leg, like a hinge, from the knee. Breathe in and place the leg back down, engaging the hamstring slightly. Make sure that you don't kick out or thump your

feet down. Your feet should be softly pointed. Repeat the movement
10 times.

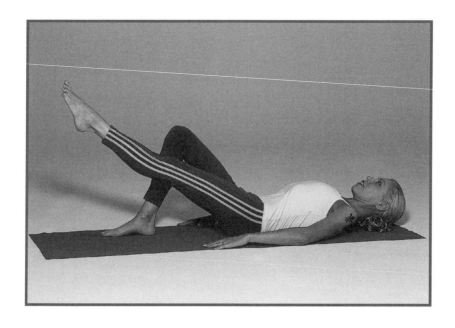

Abdominal Exercise 2

This next exercise is the same idea in reverse. Instead of extending the leg out, the knee comes up into your chest but not too high up and the leg returns to the floor. As you breathe out and place your foot back on the floor, the stomach pulls up and in. This enables a connection to be made between your navel and spine. Alternate the exercise 10 times. Don't bring your leg in so far that you feel your hip pinching.

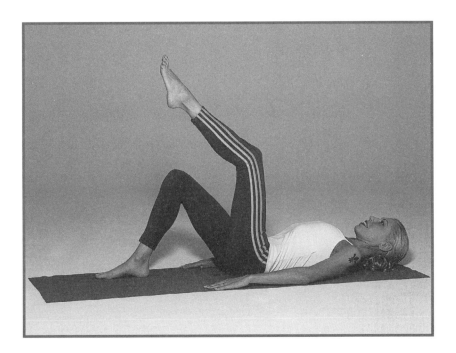

Abdominal Exercise 3

For the final abdominal exercise in this sequence, lie down on your back as before, but with your legs in a small v-shaped position. This exercise focuses on the inside thigh as well as the lower abdominal muscles.

Breathe out and extend one leg. Concentrate on your inner thigh as well as your abdominals. Bring your navel into the spine as you extend your leg. When you alternate legs, make sure you extend them the same width apart. Make sure your hips are level. You don't want one leg to be longer than the other. Don't let the weight of your quad or your thigh take over the movement. Do 10 repetitions in total.

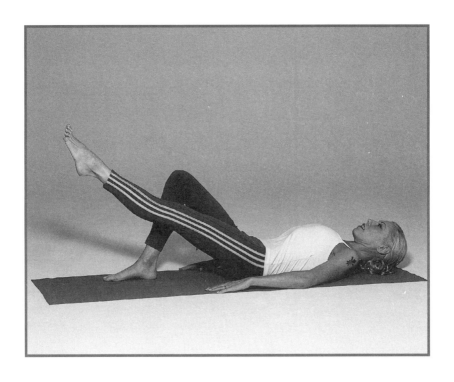

Leg Lifts

Start in the same position as the previous exercises, with both knees bent. Extend your left leg along the ground. Breathing out, lift your left leg off the floor until it is level with the right knee. At the top of the lift, flex your foot, breathe in and breathe out as you lower. Do 10 repetitions on each leg.

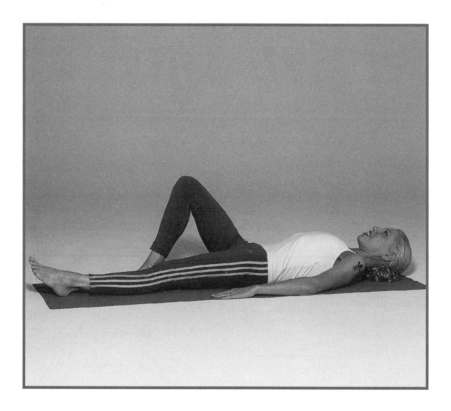

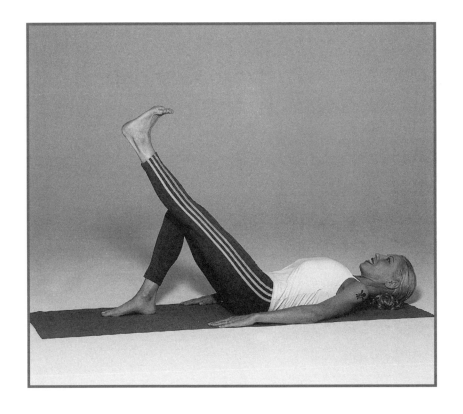

The Exercises

Hip Lengthening

This exercise helps to keep the hips mobile. Lie flat on the floor with both legs straight in front of you; flex your feet up towards you. Have your hands on your hips. Make sure that your head doesn't drop back. It is important not to arch your back – to avoid this, focus on your stomach and spine softening into the floor.

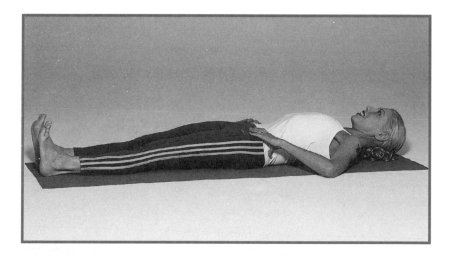

Breathing out, push one heel out further than the other, to facilitate liberation through the hip socket. Alternate legs and repeat the exercise five times on each.

Leg Circles

This is another exercise for lubricating the hips, but it also stretches out the hamstrings and exercises the stomach.

Lie down in the same position as before, with both legs straight along the floor and your hands resting on your hips. Bend one leg and lift it so that it reaches a right angle with your hip. You should be able, eventually, to do this without straining your back or neck. Rotate your leg in 10 small circles in each direction to mobilize the hip socket. Keep the circles quite small because you don't want either hip to come up off the mat. Think of the working hip as being weighted down onto the mat. Then bend the leg in and slowly lower it down.

Do five to ten circles in each direction, and then repeat the exercise with the other leg. Think of the working hip dropping into the floor. This exercise may be difficult if your hamstrings are too tight. It is also quite difficult to extend the leg comfortably to the ceiling, so build up slowly.

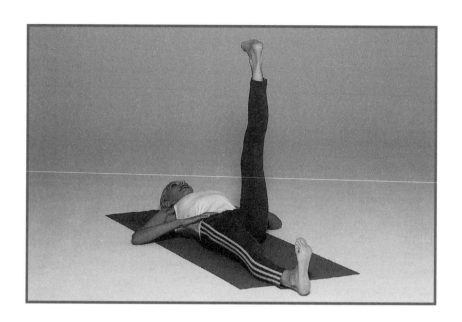

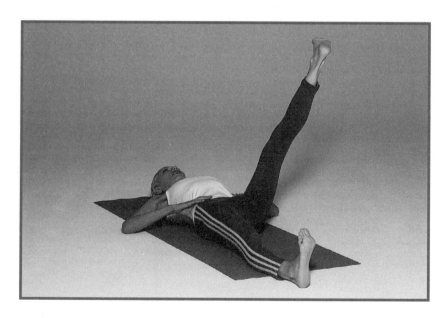

Pilates Over 50

Abdominal Curls

At this point in your routine, repeat the same *Abdominal Curls* as before (see pages 86–90) to work your centre.

＊　＊　＊

The feet are a neglected part of the body. People often complain about foot cramp when they are exercising. It is important to keep your feet relaxed and not tense. Whenever the exercises call for flexed feet, flex them gently – stretching out from your heel then pulling the top of your foot back as far as you can without straining.

Foot Exercise

Doing this exercise every day helps to strengthen the muscles in the ankles and feet. Use a blue, medium-strength Dynaband to help you.

Sit with your leg out in front of you, either on the floor or using a gym bench. Flex your foot up, working through the arch and keeping your ankle in neutral. It is important that you don't let your ankle wiggle from side to side as you use the Dynaband to pull your toes back. Don't claw your toes like a budgie on a perch. Try to bring all the toes forward and backward at the same time. Don't lock your knee into the floor. Do between six and eight repetitions on each foot.

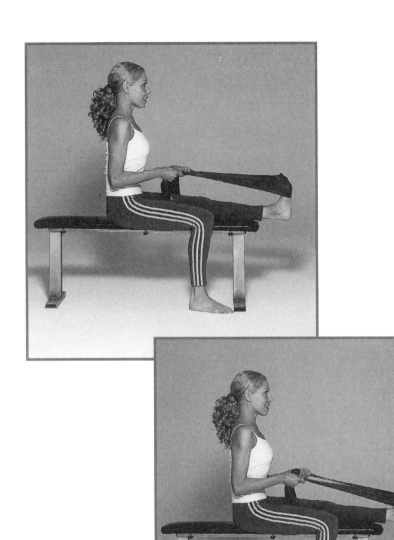

Doming

Doming helps to prepare for the standing exercises. It gives a firm base on which to stand. It's best to dome with bare feet so you can feel a good contact with the floor.

Place your heel on the mat and spread your toes evenly as the ball of your foot comes to rest on the ground. It is like resting the palm of your hand on the table and spreading out the fingers as they flatten down.

When you have firm contact with the floor, draw up the arch of your foot and create a dome between the toes and the heel. I like to imagine that there is chewing gum under the ball of my foot helping to keep it stuck to the floor even though the arch of my foot is raised up. Dome 10 times with each foot.

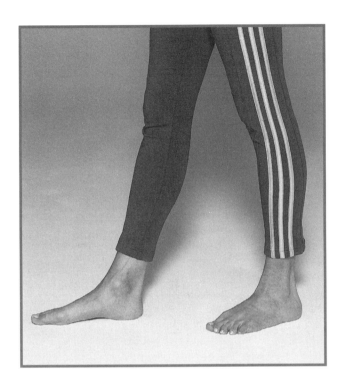

 Watchpoint: Try and work all your toes evenly.
Keep your weight over your big toe and don't roll
your foot out.

* * *

The next five exercises warm up and mobilize the shoulders and upper
body, as well as focusing on a positive posture and integrated abdominal
strength.

Arm Circles (single)

This exercise improves the mobility of the clavicle in the shoulder joint. Obey all the rules of perfect posture: your feet should be relaxed and placed hip-width apart. The weight of your body should be evenly balanced on both legs, making sure that you do not lean forwards or backwards. Relax and lengthen your toes as if they are softening into sand. Your stomach should be tucked in – feel your centre of gravity in your tailbone.

Make sure your arms are relaxed by your side by having your middle finger stretching down the outside of your thigh. Place your hands just slightly in front of you. Like your pelvis, your head should be in neutral. I imagine my head is the blossom sitting at the top of a plant: relaxed, balanced, light. Release your knees.

Once you have worked your way into this perfect standing posture – relaxed but alert to your body – circle each arm individually, four times in each direction. It is a slow and controlled movement: the circles are always just in front of your body. Don't rock back and forth. You will know that your arms are in the correct position if you can always see behind your elbow in your periphery vision. That way your body won't twist.

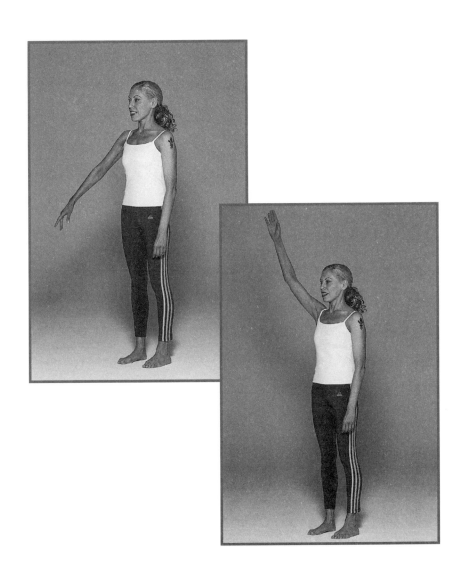

Arm Circles (double)

This is the same exercise as above, except that you rotate both arms at the same time, four times in each direction.

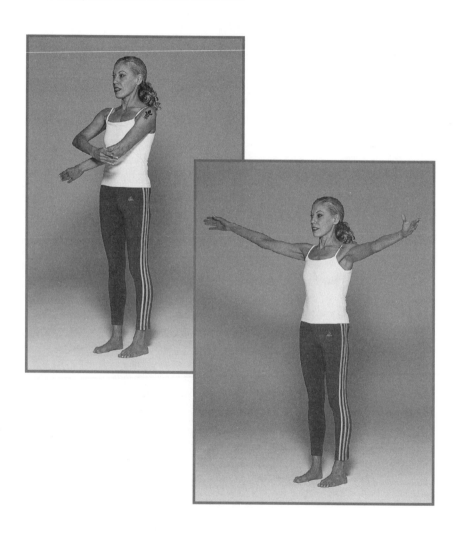

Warm-up for Shoulders and Back

This will improve your postural awareness. Again, stand with bare feet to get better contact with the floor.

Make sure you are maintaining a perfect posture (see above). Then exhale and stretch one arm to the ceiling while the other arm gently reaches behind you. There should be no movement in your feet, pelvis, upper back or neck. Alternate between each arm 10 times.

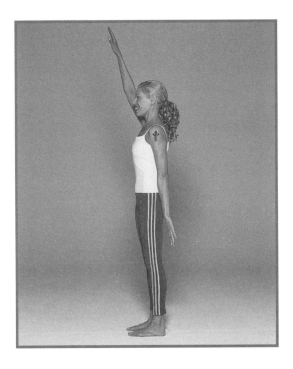

Slicing

For this fourth exercise in the sequence, stand in the same upright posture as before, making sure your feet aren't gripping and that your buttocks aren't tense.

Straighten both your arms and bring them in front of you, with the tips of the little fingers touching. Then, on the exhalation, make a slicing motion upwards and out towards the corners of the room. Your arms should stay straight the whole time.

When you have sliced 10 times you can add a diagonal variation. As you slice, gently twist your body round, so that your head follows. You will feel a stretch across your chest and your shoulders loosening up.

These exercises are about coordination and rhythm. Your arms are working together: they begin and end at the same point. You don't want one arm to begin before the other.

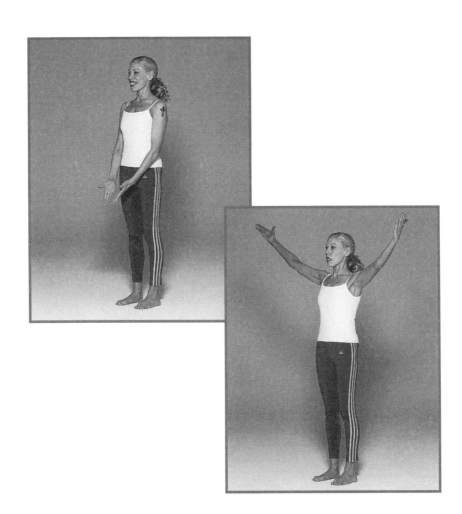

 Watchpoint: Try to resist the tendency in these exercises towards locking the elbows. All your joints are in line but not locked: the shoulders, the elbows, the wrist, all your fingers.

Brushing

Check again that you are obeying all the same rules about good posture, then raise your left arm behind your left ear, stretch it up to the crown of your head, and then away to the side – so that your arm reaches out to the same point it did when slicing. Your palm should brush the side of your ear, as if you're trying to brush it away to the side of the room. Do 10 repetitions, alternating each side.

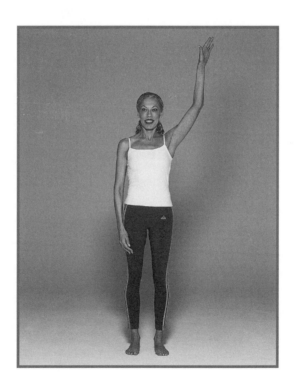

Watchpoint: To maintain a good posture, the key is making sure your arm doesn't go behind you. You will know if it does because your weight will shift back and forth, your stomach will protrude, your bottom stick out, and your back arch.

Side Stretch (arms)

This is good to do after the arm exercises because it releases the spine from side to side.

Stand up straight in perfect posture. Stretch slowly but fully from side to side, alternating each arm. Don't move your hips. Repeat the movement 10 times, again, alternating from side to side.

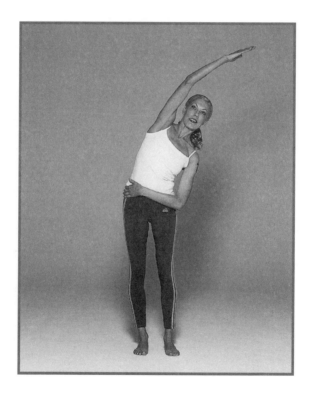

Side Lift

Lie down on your side with your elbow directly under your shoulder and your palm flat on the floor. Keep your legs in a straight line and have your ankles crossed.

Keeping your shoulder and elbow in line, breathe out and lift yourself up, pushing down through the supporting arm. The other arm lifts up to a right angle with your shoulder. Hold this position for a few seconds, and then breathe in and relax. Do 10 repetitions on each side to give a strong and toned waist.

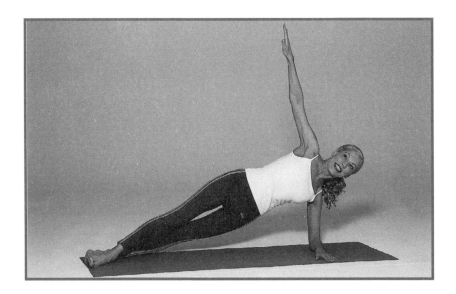

Watchpoint: Correct breathing is vital to control

the strain of this tricky exercise.

Triceps Lift

Although you are targeting the muscles in the backs of your arms, this is also a full body exercise. It works the back and upper body, and stabilizes the pelvis. It should be possible for everyone to lift their own body weight, and this exercise will help achieve that goal.

Sit with your legs stretched out in front of you, leaning on your arms behind. Your palms should rest on the floor and point towards you. Personally, I start with my elbows bent because I have very long arms. Breathe out and push up with both arms simultaneously. Breathe in again and lower yourself to the floor. Repeat this 10 times.

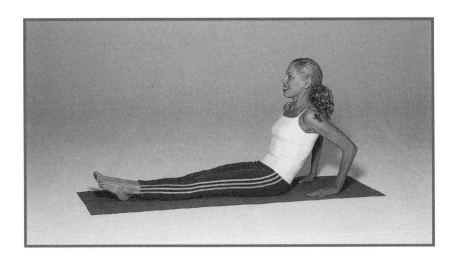

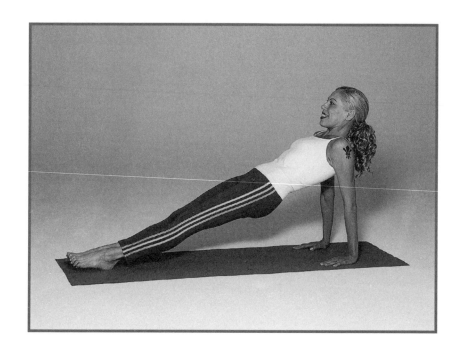

Side Stretch

Now the core body work continues. Lie down on your side with your lower arm stretched out along the ground above your head, in line with your body, palm down. The other hand is placed lightly out in front of you, to help your balance. You may need a towel between your ear and your shoulder to keep your neck comfortable and lengthened.

There is a temptation to let the hips rock forward in this position, so check that your hips are stacked one above the other and that your pelvis is level. Look down your body (without moving your head) to check that you can see your feet. That way you will know that they are not too far behind you.

Breathing out, lift your legs about 10cm off the floor. Imagine your legs floating up. Your feet should be gently flexed and the backs of your legs perfectly straight. The energy pushes out through the heels as you lift up 10 times on each side. As you go place your legs down each time, breathe in.

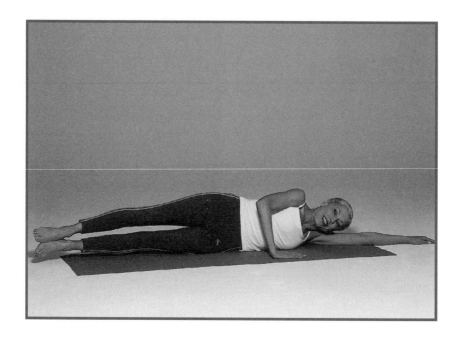

 Watchpoint: As with all the exercises, do not lock your knees. They should be lengthening away and slightly released.

Press-ups

Now you're ready to continue with your upper body toning and
strengthening. Kneel down on a mat or a towel and make a square with
your body: your knees should be directly under your hips and your hands
under your shoulders – just wider than shoulder-width apart, with the
palms flat and fingers pointing away from you. (An alternative is to have
one hand crossed over the other.) Keeping your head in line, gently tip
your weight forwards. Your feet should stay flat on the floor.

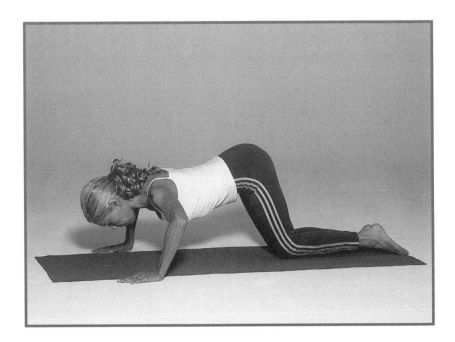

Inhaling, bend your elbows and press your head, shoulders and chest towards the floor. Then raise yourself up again, slowly, on the exhalation. It helps the concentration to focus on the same spot on the floor throughout. You can build up to between 25 and 50 repetitions of this exercise.

As a variation – to make the exercise slightly harder – you can cross your ankles and lift your feet up off the ground. This tips the weight further over the arms, thus working your upper body more effectively. However, at no point should you arch your back or lose the alignment from the crown of the head through to your tailbone.

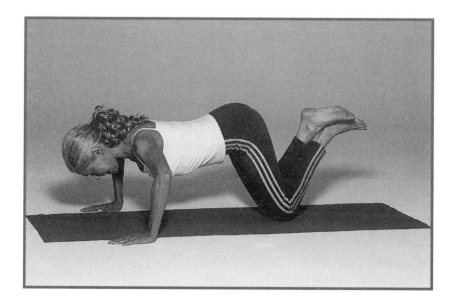

Watchpoint: Don't arch your back and make sure you keep your stomach tucked in.

Watchpoint: Keep your head in a natural position – neither forwards nor backwards.

Dips

Dips are sometimes difficult for women because they often lack strength in the backs of their arms.

Place a chair against a wall for support, or use a secure bench. Resting your hands on the edge of the seat, about a shoulder-width apart, place your knees in line with your feet. If they aren't in line, then you won't be using the correct muscle groups for this exercise: the thighs will take over from the backs of the arms.

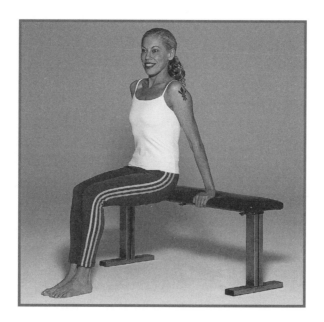

Once you're in the correct position, bend your elbows as you breathe in and slide down the front of the chair; then, as you breathe out, push back up to the starting position. Aim to build up to 20 to 30 repetitions, making sure that you slide your bottom straight down and not forward. That way you support all the weight with your arms and not your thighs.

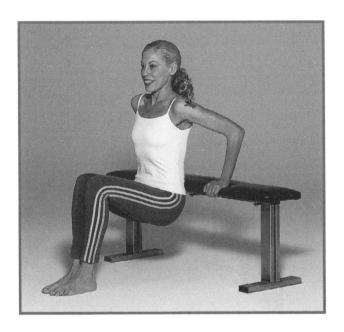

 Watchpoint: Don't start by doing 20 to 30 repetitions! This is a tough exercise and it takes time to reach this point. Build up slowly.

The Exercises

When you are strong enough, repeat the *Press-up* exercise again followed by the *Dips*. It is more effective to build up to 20 of each exercise and then repeat, rather than do single sets of 30 of each exercise.

Straight Arm Side Lifts

NB: This exercise is very advanced and should not be attempted by beginners or anyone with back or joint problems.

The ability to lift your own body weight is important because it strengthens your joints. Only about 10 per cent of my clients can do this exercise.

Start in the same position as the *Side Lift* (page 115), but with a straight supporting arm. Make a small bend with the top of your arm and push yourself up, creating the right-angled triangle shape beneath your raised body. Do not distort your pelvis. The most common error is to sink into the supporting shoulder: you should keep your arm straight. Do 10 lifts on each side.

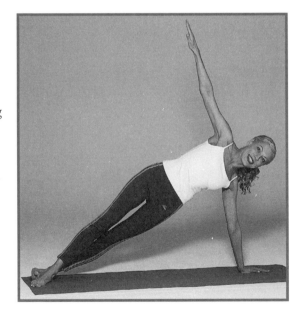

Full Press-ups

NB: This exercise is very advanced and should not be attempted by beginners or anyone with back or joint problems.

There is no point in doing full press-ups if you can't keep your navel tucked into your spine. Do not attempt full press-ups if you have thoracic scoliosis.

Place your hands under your shoulders – just wider than shoulder-width apart – but this time, your legs are out straight. Don't pinch your shoulder blades. Your weight should be evenly and widely spread over your hands, which face forwards. Breathe in as you go down and out as you go up. Start with eight repetitions, and build up the numbers from there.

Make sure the energy goes back over the heels and you have equal pressure over both hands so as not to favour one side or the other.

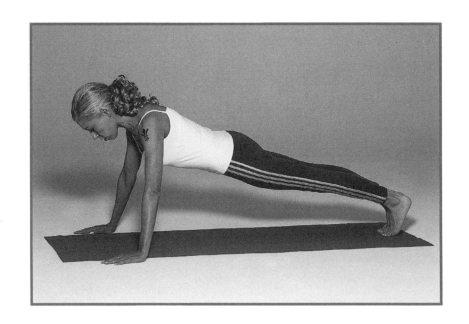

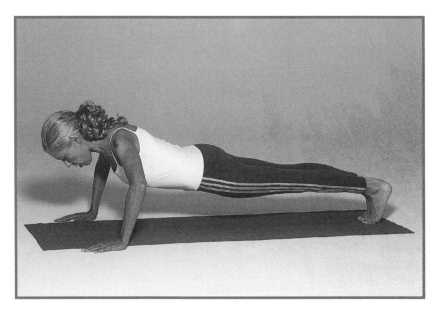

Shoulder Stretch

After this upper body strengthening, it is important to stretch out your shoulders. I usually stand up for this exercise, although it can be done sitting down.

Holding your arms up in front of your face, cross one over the other and clasp your hands together. Then gently push your elbows to the ceiling and feel your shoulders stretching apart. As you raise your arms, keep your shoulders down and hold this position for a count of 10. Repeat this stretch four times, alternating arms.

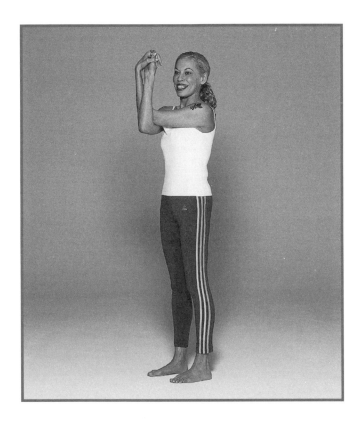

* * *

Before I move on to using ankle weights I do the hip roll sequence to
mobilize my spine. The reason I put it in here is because now I've really
focused on my centre, and it is vital not to allow the weight of the leg do
the work – the abdominal muscles should be the instigators of these
movements.

The Exercises

Hip Roll (legs crossed)

This three-part mobilization exercise for the spine helps to release your back. It also stretches out the lower back and hips.

For the first in the hip roll sequence, you should lie in the same position as for the *Pelvic Tilt* (page 77), but with one leg crossed over the other. The other foot is firmly on the floor. Stretch your arms out horizontally just below shoulder level, with your palms flat on the floor.

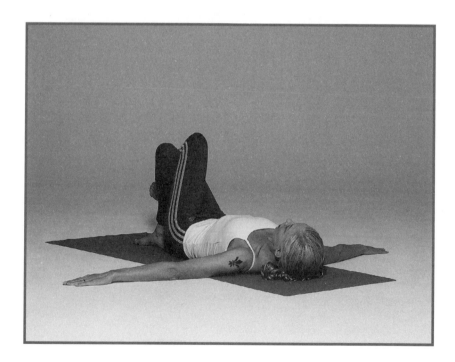

Breathe out to execute a diagonal stretch through the spine. Your legs go one way and your head goes the other. Breathe in and move back to the centre; breathe out and reverse the stretch. As you breathe out, take a gentle turn towards your lower leg, with your head looking in the opposite direction. Never pivot so far round that your shoulders are tempted to lift up off the floor. Turn 10 times in this position before swapping legs and twisting again another 10 times.

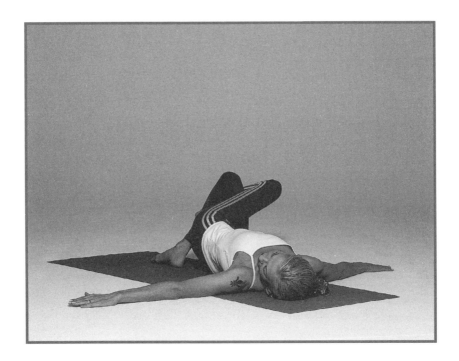

Hip Roll (both legs)

This is a more difficult exercise than the first version. Your legs are uncrossed and are bent into your chest. Your knees are in line with your hips and your feet are relaxed. As you breathe out, your legs go one way, your head goes the other way, and your stomach remains in. Breathe in and come back to the centre.

The most important part of this exercise is that at no point does either shoulder blade leave the mat. Your knees should stay together as you move from side to side – this way one leg won't get longer than the other. It is very natural as you turn from side to side for the top knee to shorten, but try to avoid this tendency.

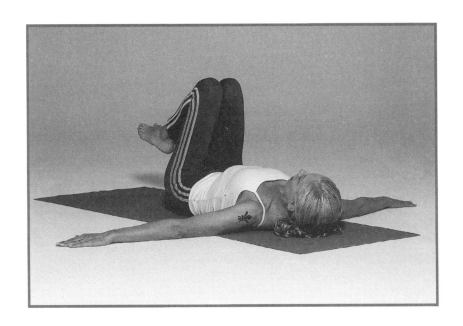

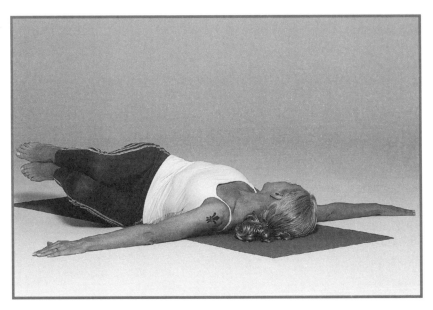

Hip Roll (single leg)

Do this last version only twice – once with the right leg on top, once with the left, then repeat.

Start in the same position as before, with your knees into your chest and your arms beside you, below shoulder height. Then place your left leg flat on the floor. As you breathe out, twist the top leg over, then breathe in and come back to centre. Your lower leg stays flat on the floor. Your upper leg starts out bent, but then, at the full extent of the roll, straighten it out so that it points away nearly at right angles with your hips. Then do the same with the other leg as you roll the other way.

I do the next selection of exercises at least three times a week with ankle weights. If I'm going to do them more often, I don't always use the weights. I never use more than a 1kg weight, because I am toning and my muscles should be lengthening and strengthening, not getting bigger.

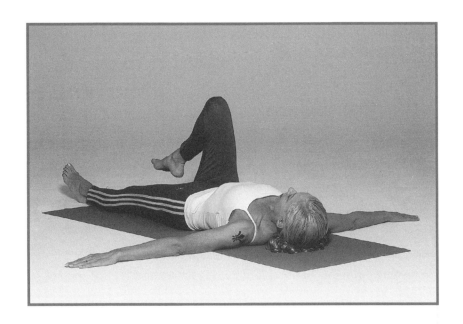

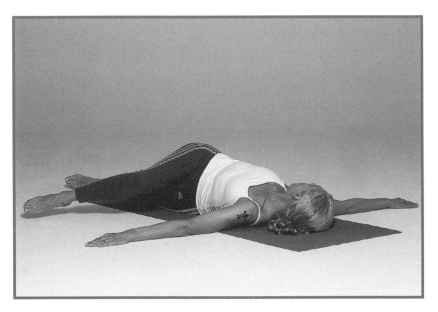

When I do these exercises I always focus on working from the centre. Because you are working on the side think of the same principles that you will have used in the sequence of side stretches and side lifts. Exactly the same muscles are working but you then include the legs afterwards. Don't just heave away at your leg without focusing on your centre.

There is a huge range of exercises for the legs, but I've found the ones included here to be the most effective and the most efficient, and my clients agree with me. At the end of this sequence there is a selection of leg stretches. I cannot emphasize too strongly that you *must* do these stretches after the sequence so that your muscles don't contract and get tighter. If you are running out of time, make sure you do these stretches even if it means leaving out the rest of the mat work programme.

Inside Thigh Toner

If you do these exercises every day as part of your exercise routine, your thighs will never be flabby.

Lie down on your side, either with your hand supporting your head or your arm completely flat and a towel between your arm and your ear. Your other arm is resting, palm down, on the floor for support.

Bend your top leg in front of you. The lower leg (the one that will do all the work) is placed slightly forward of your body, with your foot gently flexed. Make sure your leg is straight by pulling up the muscles through the inside of the knee and thighs. This does not mean your knee is locked – just fully extended. This way you will be working the thighs and not the ankles and feet.

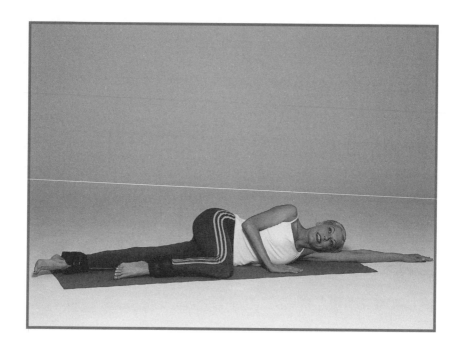

Breathing out, lift your lower leg so that it lengthens away as it rises up. You should be lengthening and strengthening your muscles rather than having them contracted and tight. Your foot is flexed and parallel. As you lift and breathe out, your stomach pulls in, just as in the earlier side stretches and lift exercises (pages 96–119). Your energy flows through your heel from your inside thigh. Lower your leg. Do 10 repetitions on each side.

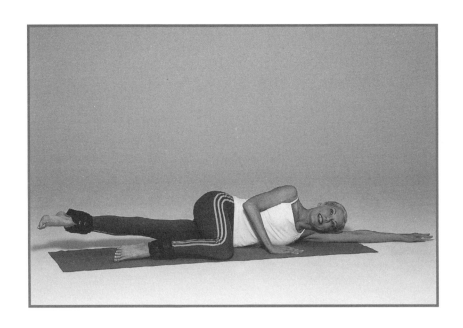

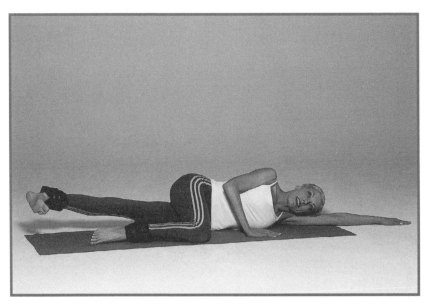

You can change the position of your feet after 10 repetitions: they start out flexed and parallel; then they are pointed and turned out with the leg rotating in the hip socket. Then add the third variation. Lift your underneath, working, leg, which you bend and straighten 10 times before lowering. The foot is flexed and parallel as in the first exercise.

 Watchpoint: In all the leg exercises, your stomach is the instigator of the movement.

Buttock and Outer Thigh Toner

Start in the same position as before, only this time your bottom leg is bent in front of you, while your top leg is straight and flexed, slightly in front of the top hip. Make sure your back doesn't arch.

Your top leg starts the exercise at hip height. Breathing in, lift the leg up about 20cm. Don't turn your toes towards the ceiling; your foot should face forwards, gently flexed. When you breathe out, bring your top leg forward until it is in line with the underneath bent knee. Breathe in and return the leg to its original position. Do not rest between your 10 repetitions: your leg should never touch the floor.

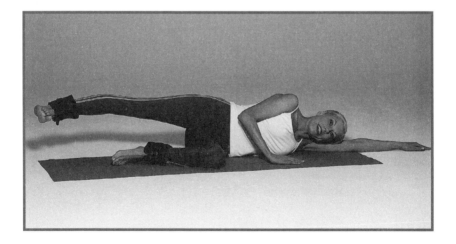

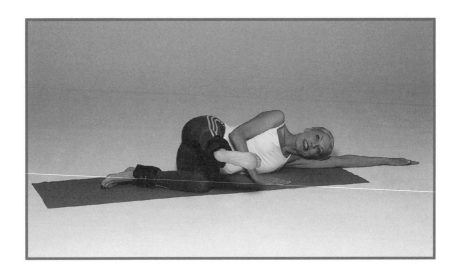

Watchpoint: As you breathe out and pull your leg forward, don't swing it. Think of your leg as resistance, so that it is your stomach that is bringing your leg forward and back as you tone the back of your thigh. Your hip stays back; your stomach stays in.

Buttock and Outer Thigh Toner (version 2)

The second buttock exercise continues from the previous one. Don't rest between the two exercises. When you have completed the 10 repetitions on one side, continue holding your leg in line with the other knee. Then breathe out as you bend and straighten the working leg. The emphasis is not on the bend but on the squeeze. If the bend is too big, then your calves would be doing the work rather than your bottom.

Once you have done 10 repetitions of the squeeze, change sides and do the sequence of the two exercises again. If you find the exercise particularly strenuous, alternate sides.

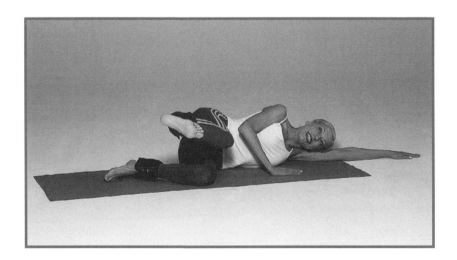

Standing Calf Stretch

Stand up straight and tall, following the perfect posture rules (see page 106). Then take a step forward with your right leg, so that it is slightly bent in front of you. Your left leg remains straight behind you, although you are leaning forward. Keeping your heel down on your back leg ensures the stretch works properly. Do not bounce – hold this position firmly for 30 seconds and repeat twice on each leg.

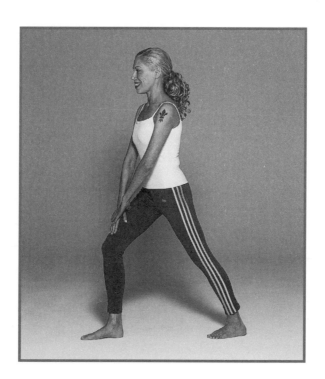

Seated Gluteal Stretch

Sitting on the floor, stretch your left leg out in front of you. Cross your right foot over the outside of the left knee, keeping the right hand on the floor. Bend the left knee to bring your left foot towards your right buttock.

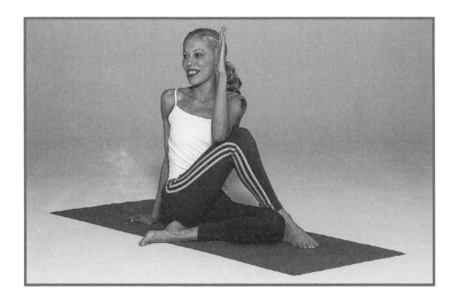

With your left hand, hold your right knee and gently ease it into your chest. Then rotate your body around to the right, and feel the stretch through your buttock. Your bent leg is in front of you. Repeat four times, alternating legs.

Seated Hamstring Stretches

Sitting on the floor, with the soles of your feet together and your knees apart, take hold of your left foot and take a diagonal stretch to the side ensuring that you do not lean into the stretch. Hold for 10 seconds and change legs. Do this twice on each side, stretching out the back of your knees as fully as possible. The more you flex your foot, the greater the stretch through the calf, hamstring and inside thigh.

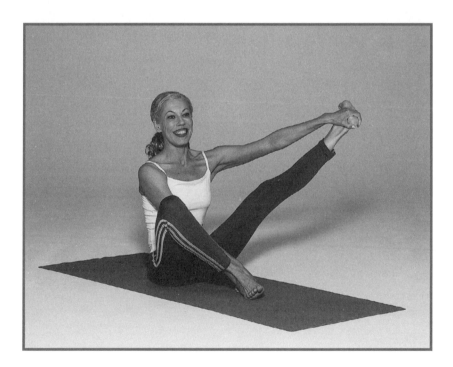

When you have repeated this twice on each side, focus on your balance, and using core abdominal strength, stretch out and hold both legs for 10 seconds, and then repeat the movement.

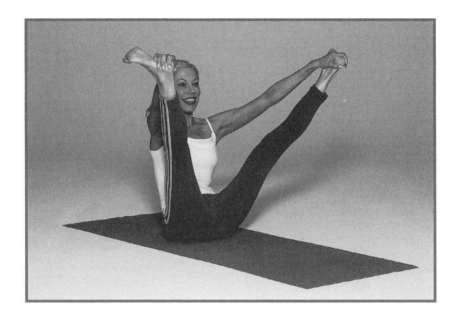

You need good balance for these exercises, so if your abdominal muscles are weak or your hamstrings too tight, concentrate on the alternate leg stretch first. You don't want to fall backwards and crack your head!

Quadriceps Stretch

Kneel down on your right leg, keeping your back straight. Then extend your left leg, making sure that your heel is always in front of your knee. Pull your stomach in and lean back slightly, making sure you don't make an arch. Hold this posture for 30 seconds, and repeat it twice for each leg.

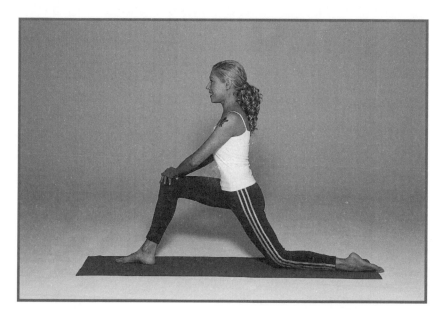

 Watchpoint: If you feel any pain in your knees, STOP at once.

To make this exercise more challenging, take hold of your back foot with both hands and draw it towards your bottom.

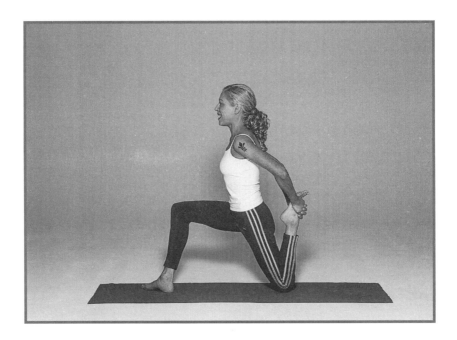

Standing Hamstring Stretch

Start standing upright with both legs parallel, and then place one leg on a chair or gym bench. Your foot should be flexed. Keep your standing leg slightly bent and your stomach tucked in. Your neck and shoulders should be relaxed, and your hips level.

Slide your hands down your raised leg towards your outstretched foot. This will make you feel a wonderful stretch in your hamstring between your knee and hip. Hold this posture for 30 seconds and then repeat twice for each leg.

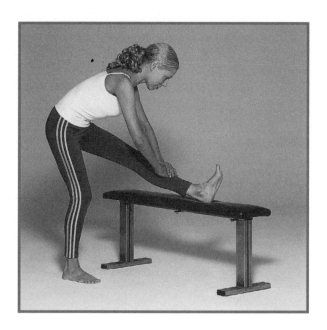

Pilates Over 50

Inner Thigh Stretch

Sit on the floor with your back straight. Hold your ankles and keep the soles of your feet together. Then curl forwards, relax your shoulders, and let your knees drop out to the side. With every exhalation, feel your knees sinking further towards the ground. Then breathe into the new space you've created in your hips. Do four repetitions of this exercise, holding the position for 30 seconds each time.

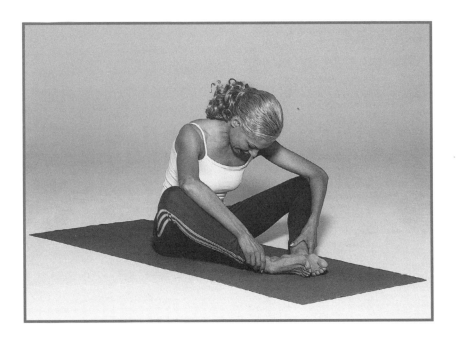

* * *

I like to do my back strengthening exercises near the end of my programme because they all focus on working from a strong centre. At no time should you feel the lumbar spine – the lower back – tightening or shortening. You're working on increasing the flexibility of your spine on flexion and extension. Always remember that the abdominals are the motivator for these exercises.

These are the back exercises I do when I am not in my studio, because they don't require special equipment. These back exercises are very effective. However, it is only by using the specialized Pilates equipment in my Body Maintenance studio that I have been able to make my back as strong as it is. You can achieve a lot without specialized equipment, but it takes longer.

Complicated Cat Stretch

This is great for strengthening and stretching your shoulders, upper back, and chest.

Kneel down and make a square with your body – the same shape as for the press-ups (page 121). Place your knees under your hips with your hands under your shoulders. Relax your feet.

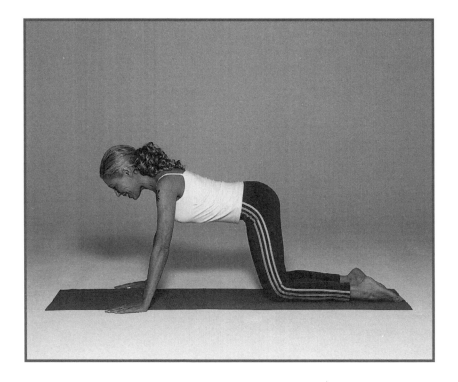

Breathing out, pull your stomach in, curl your back like a cat, and tuck your chin into your chest. Your bottom sinks down towards your heels. Breathing in, bend your elbows so that you stretch your chest down towards the floor. Coming back up again, raise your head slightly and slowly, making sure that you don't feel a crunch in the back of your neck.

Breathe out as your stomach contracts into your spine. Breathe in to release. Repeat the whole process 10 times. At the end, sit back on your heels to stretch out your back.

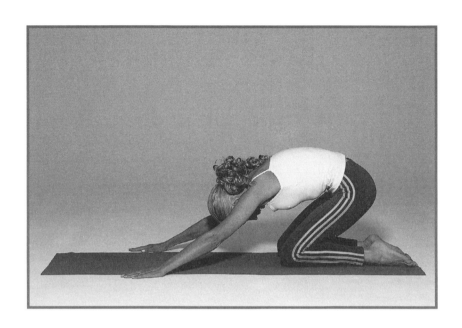

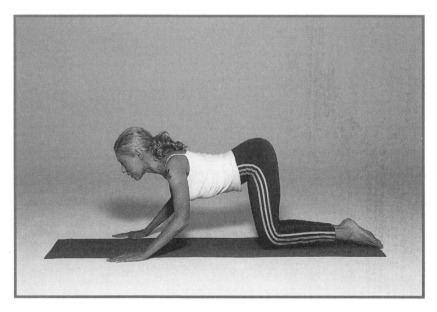

Back Strengthening

This is for lengthening as well as strengthening. Lie down on your stomach with your feet flat and relaxed. Your arms are pointed slightly forwards with your hands just wider than shoulder-width apart.

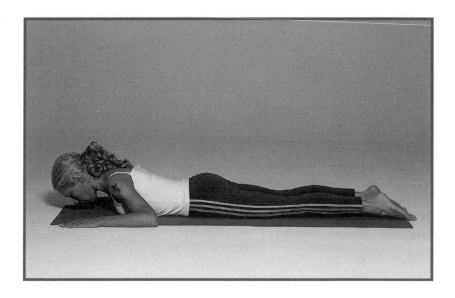

As you breathe out, raise your chest up and gently press your hips and elbows into the floor and pull your stomach in. To keep your neck long, look down at the floor. Then gently lift your head up, but keep your eyes focused on the same point. Make sure you keep your feet firmly on the floor. Breathe in and relax down again. Engaging the abdominals will strengthen your back and improve your posture.

When you're lifting up, you might find it helpful to imagine that the crown of your head is going forwards, towards the wall in front of you. Don't lift your head up to the ceiling. There should be very little pressure on your hands – it is your stomach muscles that are doing all the lifting. Your hands should be relaxed. Repeat this five times, with your elbows remaining on the floor. Then try straightening your elbows for a further five repetitions.

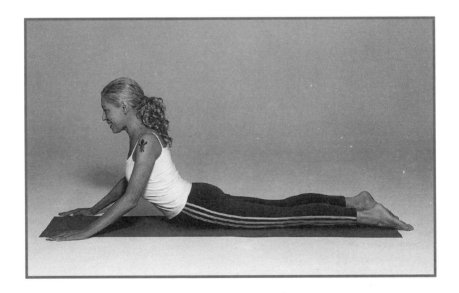

Watchpoint: When you breathe out, your stomach goes into the spine. At no point should your shoulders scrunch up towards your ears, nor should you lift yourself so high that your lower back tightens. Think of the abdominals flattening towards the spine as the body leaves the floor.

Alternate Arm and Leg Stretch for the Back

The idea of this exercise is to do a diagonal stretch that strengthens and mobilizes the big back muscle between the base of one shoulder blade and the top of the opposite buttock.

Lying on your stomach, imagine yourself to be in the shape of a starfish. Your arms are slightly wider apart than your shoulders. Look down at the floor. Your legs are comfortably apart and rotated outwards slightly. This is their relaxed natural position.

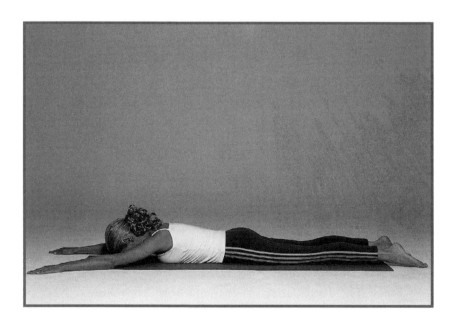

Breathing out, let your left leg and your right arm float off the ground. You should be able to feel your stomach doing all the work. Breathe in as you lower again, and then exhale as you change sides.

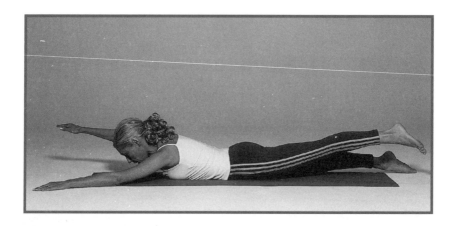

Your stomach is tucked in and your tailbone drops. Don't grip your bottom as you breathe. Again, keep your legs straight and your shoulders relaxed. Your arms and legs should lift to the same height. Do 10 repetitions, alternating sides.

Watchpoint: Don't shorten your neck, grip your bottom or lift your arm or leg too high. Think of lengthening rather than lifting your limbs.

The Swan

Maintain the starfish position. All the same rules about posture and movement apply here as in the previous exercise.

As you breathe out, simultaneously lift both arms and legs to the same height. Keep looking down at the floor throughout. Pull your stomach into your spine until you feel your tailbone drop.

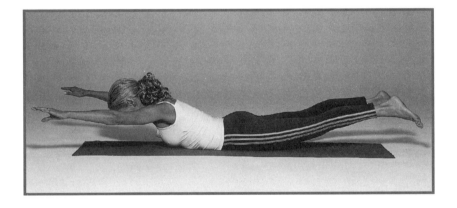

Watchpoint: As your stomach goes in, don't grip your bottom.

Watchpoint: Keep your legs straight; the exercise won't be effective with bent legs. Keep your shoulders relaxed.

The remaining few exercises are some alternatives to press-ups and dips. I've also included the four exercises that you can see demonstrated on a gym bench. I do these on a barrel when I'm at my studio, because this allows you to have a greater range of movement. But a gym bench is just as effective, so long as you make sure your back doesn't arch. The *Arms Opening* and the *Arm Circles* are two of the most essential exercises to avoid the ugly signs of ageing – the rounded shoulders and the forward pointing neck. The point is to increase the flexibility and mobility in the shoulder joint. It is about realigning the upper body, the neck and the shoulders, so you have the upright standing posture of someone a third your age.

Biceps Curl

Stand in perfect posture holding a 2kg weight in each hand. Breathing in, bend your arm up to shoulder level. Breathing out, straighten your arm back to waist level. Don't rock back and forth as you do this. Repeat this exercise 15 times with each arm.

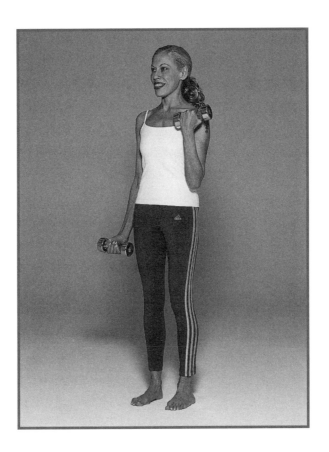

Triceps Press

Use a chair to make a square with your body. Place your right hand and knee on the chair and keep your left leg straight on the ground. Your neck is in line with the rest of your body. Holding a 2kg weight, lift your right arm as high as you can, keeping your elbow bent at a right angle, without twisting your body. On the exhalation, straighten the arm out behind you. After a pause, bend your arm back again. Repeat this exercise 15 times on each arm.

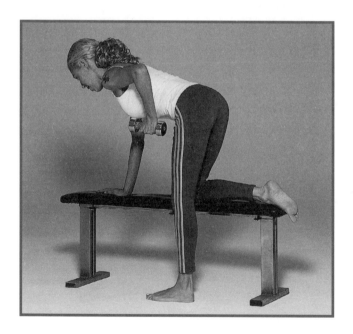

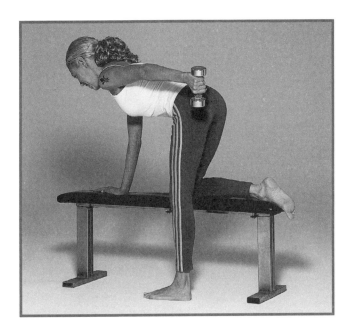

Alternate this exercise with the *Biceps Curl*. The entire sequence should be 15 Biceps Curls on each arm, then 15 Triceps Presses on each arm, all of which is repeated twice more.

✳ ✳ ✳

These last four exercises are for toning the arms and shoulders. They remedy tight, rounded shoulders, a forward pointing neck, and a tight upper back. In my Pilates studio I do these exercises on specialized equipment. In the gym I use a bench. I make sure that my back does not arch at any point. Using 1kg weights on each arm helps to stretch and mobilize and achieve perfect alignment of the upper back and neck. Slightly heavier weights can only be used when you have achieved the necessary shoulder mobility so there is no discomfort in the joint.

Arms Opening

Lie on your back with your arms raised above your chest. It helps to imagine that you are a tulip: your arms open out like petals as you breathe out. When you breathe in again, bring your arms together above your chest. Your elbows are never straight – they are curled. Open and close 10 times.

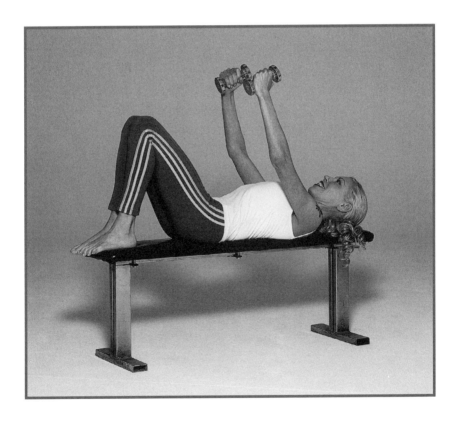

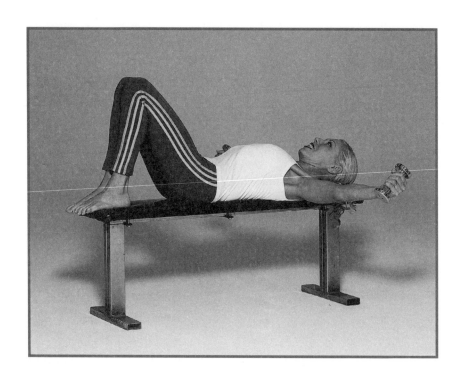

Backstroke

Lie in the same position as for the previous exercise with your arms above your chest. Your palms should face forward and point towards the wall in front of you. Your shoulders are relaxed. As you breathe out, one arm goes behind you; the other goes down by your side. Breathe in as you reverse your arms. It is like doing backstroke. Repeat this exercise 20 times: 10 times for each arm.

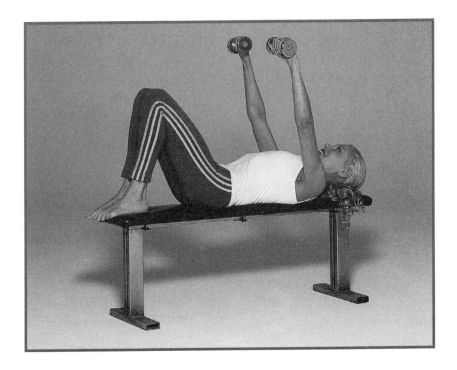

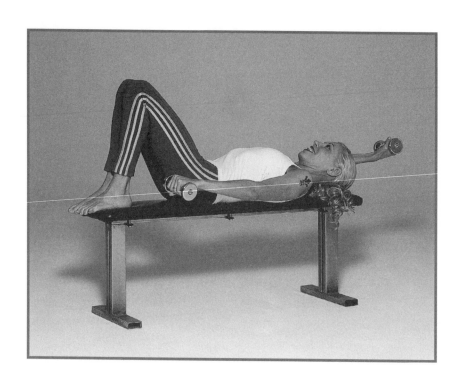

Pilates Over 50

Shoulder Stretch

Still lying on your back, holding one weight, making a diamond shape
with your elbows. As you breathe out, take the shape behind your head,
brushing past your ears, as far back as you can without your back lifting
up. Repeat this 10 times.

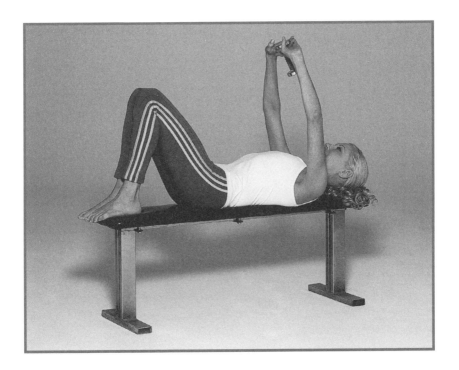

Arm Circles

Assume the same position as in the Arms Opening exercise. With your arms stretched up above you, breathe out and make a circle, so that the hands reach as far behind you as possible, then down to the floor and stretch to your feet without any arch in the lower back. Then bring your arms back and stretch them towards your hips on the inhalation. Do 10 circles one way, then 10 the other.

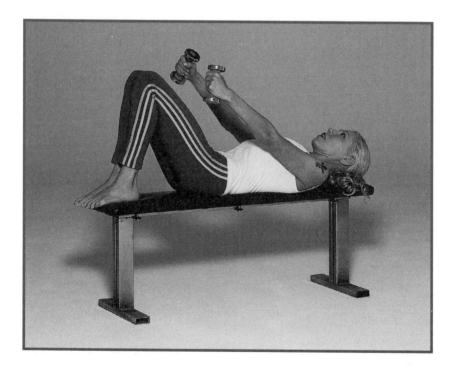

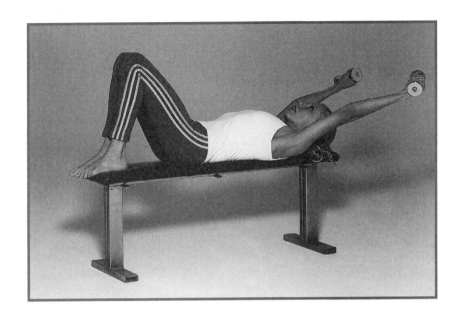

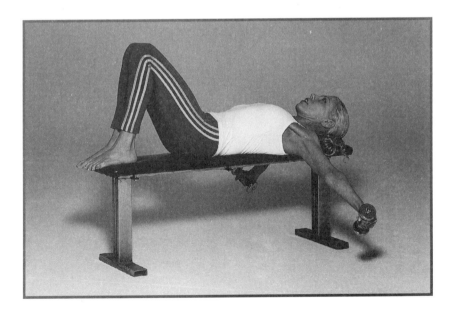

If these four arm exercises are performed correctly, they will remedy the stooping posture which comes with ageing. Remember: stand tall and straight, and keep moving forward in your life.

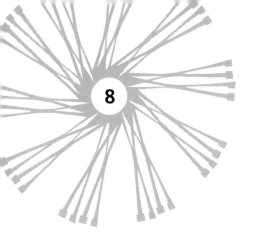

8

Case Study

I've known Janet for 10 or 12 years now and for a long time, mutual friends had been encouraging her to come to my studio and exercise. But Janet had personal trainers and all sorts of other commitments, and felt the time wasn't right. Eventually she was driven by circumstance to come to the studio around five years ago, and has been exercising here two or three times a week ever since.

Janet: I'm sixty-one years old. I've had eight pregnancies and six children, though they're not children any more. Their ages range from twenty-four to thirty-nine. Before I went to Lesley I was exercising quite a lot, having started in my mid-forties, when my children had grown up, when I realized that it wasn't quite as easy to stay as fit and slim as you can when you're young. I was encouraged to train. Then I think I probably just did too much. I was going to a gym and I used to do a lot of running and power walking – and certainly not enough stretching. I did circuits and boxercise and enjoyed it all, but I suddenly realized that I was getting a strange pain in my leg, which turned out to be quite serious sciatica. It was during treatment for this that I started to go to Lesley and Body Maintenance.

But Janet hasn't just had children and exercised. She's been an incredibly successful person. She did something that was very dynamic and challenging and which you wouldn't expect an ordinary sedentary housewife to throw herself into.

Only Lesley could ever think that a housewife mother of six was ever sedentary! I could never sit down. That's why I didn't need to exercise. In fact I had always worked as well. I was a journalist from quite a young age. I worked for national newspapers like the *Daily Mail* and for magazines. In the 1970s I worked for *Nova*, which was a deeply trendy magazine. So I was working while all the children were young. I did have help from nannies and grannies, but it was a very busy and rather competitive lifestyle. For the last fifteen years of my working life, I gave up journalism and started to run a shop selling young designers' clothes, accessories and jewellery. The shop expanded into three shops round London with business partners – selling young designers' jewellery. So that was also a busy working period. Life still seems to be busy now too, because I'm becoming a granny.

When Janet started coming to the studio, we had to do serious remedial work to restructure her body. To begin with there was a lot of work to reverse the problems with a back condition, which had brought on her sciatica. This has been ongoing. Initially Janet thought she was just going to come to me for remedial work aimed at getting her back on the treadmill. She started enjoying the work we did so much that she incorporated it into a general fitness programme. A lot of the exercises that she does are in this book. It also became clear that if she didn't come to see me regularly, her sciatica problems would flare up again. They have done, but they have been much more easily rectified due to the amount of flexibility work we incorporated into her programme.

When I first went to Lesley I was in serious trouble. I was very fortunate because my doctor sent me to a new Westminster clinic that was meant to catch back problems before they became chronic. So I saw an osteopath, a chiropractor and a physiotherapist. They told me not to do any exercise at all. Fortunately I chose to compromise and go to Lesley, who devised a very careful, limited, programme of things that I could do. Gradually the sciatica started to subside. The experts said I wouldn't be able to go running again, and wasn't swimming a much a better idea? However, I don't like the water so it wasn't a better idea for me! If I wanted to exercise in the way I had been doing, which was quite vigorously, I would have to carry on doing Pilates as well, because it enabled me to do all the other things by keeping me flexible.

I feel more stable now. I feel more balanced. Before I went to Lesley I used to trip over a lot. I'm a particularly klutzy person, so it's helped a lot with that. I was also having lower back problems – it would suddenly feel as if it was going, sometimes for no good reason or sometimes if I was over busy or tired. Pilates has helped with all of that too. Now I do a general programme that enables me to feel fitter, more balanced and more relaxed in my body, and more stretched out.

During the last two years I've been doing a lot of power walking, including a power-walking marathon through the night in aid of breast cancer research. I certainly wouldn't have been able to do that without Pilates.

Janet has a very rounded programme, and a lot of the exercises she does are included in this book. The earlier exercises I talked about, the squeezing of the towel and the pelvic floor exercises (pages 48 and 50) are absolutely vital to Janet's routine. I have included here two more exercises, not in the earlier pages: a pelvic tilt exercise (which is less advanced that the one shown on page 77) and the simple cat stretch, both of which Janet does on a weekly basis. She had to have surgery to recently – a small pelvic floor repair. Because of that we have modified her programme to included a lot more basic pelvic floor strengthening, which is very similar to the sort of exercises one would do post-pregnancy, with very successful results.

Pelvic Tilt

You may need to place a small towel behind your head. Your feet, hips and knees are all parallel, hip-width apart; your tailbone is relaxed on the mat without feeling forced down. Your shoulders are relaxed and the neck is long, and your arms lie relaxed beside you.

Without gripping your bottom, very gently tip your pelvis upwards as you breathe out; breathe in and lower back to the ground. This is a low pelvic tilt. You don't want to lift higher than your waist. You are only lifting your lower back off the ground. It's important to exhale as you lift. Breathe in, keeping your neck long, and roll all the way down.

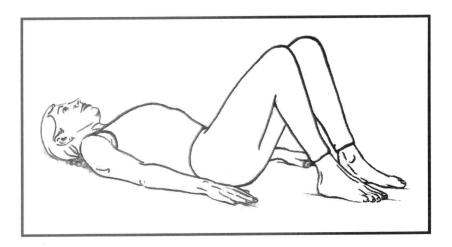

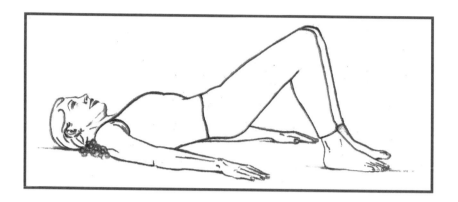

Do about 10 repetitions.

Try to get the primary curve in your lower back working to warm up the

lower back, bringing the blood supply into that area.

Simple Cat Stretch

This is done on your hands and knees. Make a square shape with your body. Keep your hands directly under your shoulders, fingers facing forwards. Your knees should be hip-width apart. If your knees feel a bit uncomfortable, just fold up a towel and put it under them. Place your feet gently on the floor and don't lock your elbows at any point. As you breathe out, drop your chin to your chest and curl your stomach into the spine. Press your upper back to the ceiling, trying not to rock back and forth. As you breathe in, your tailbone lifts towards the ceiling, your chest presses to the floor and your head gently lifts. Breathe out and reverse the position. After 10 repetitions, relax your bottom onto your heels and just breathe. This is called the 'relaxation position'.

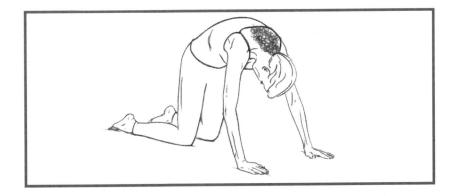

I think Pilates sounds very easy compared with a lot of fast circuit work. People think that it is dead easy and not that challenging. In fact it's incredibly difficult to do properly; I think I would not do it properly without being watched because my mind wanders onto other things. It's crucial to concentrate on the exercise, on breathing correctly, and on not tensing other parts of the body when you're focusing on a specific area. I also have very bad recall of an exercise sequence so I do have to think hard about what I'm going do next and whether I'm doing it properly! It requires a lot of commitment and concentration to do Pilates properly. But without doing Pilates I know for certain that I wouldn't be able to run, walk, leap, or even perhaps be as mobile as I am. I'm constantly amazed by some of the people I know who are a similar age to me who seem to be getting infirm – which makes me even more determined to carry on.

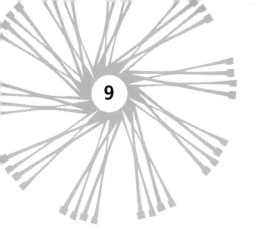

9

Conclusion

There are many reasons why each one of us exercises. For some, it has to do with physical beauty, but for many others it is about energy and quality of life. Pilates will give you a toned and flexible body no matter what your age or your circumstances. As time goes on, it will also enable you to adjust to physiological changes. You will walk with confidence, and feel leaner and taller. It will make you feel attractive and boost your self-confidence and self-esteem. The concentration required to do the exercises properly will also keep you mentally alert and agile. More importantly, it will empower you to start making small and big changes not only in your physical life, but in your mental outlook as well. Glamour is ephemeral, but physical and psychological well-being are too good to miss in the here and now.